Advance Praise to *Navi* *Restless Legs S*

"Dr. Spector articulates the ongoing shift in RLS management away from dopamine agonists with their grave long-term risks to the importance of evaluating and aggressively supplementing iron. This book confronts the complexities of this condition but is eloquently written in a way understandable to a wide audience when updated information about this disease could not be more needed."

—**Andy Berkowski**, MD, ReLACS Health, Ann Arbor, MI

"Navigating Life with Restless Legs Syndrome, authored by sleep-trained neurologist Dr. Andrew Spector, stands out as a compassionate and comprehensive guide within the American Academy of Neurology's Neurology Now Books series. Patient-centric at its core, Dr. Spector skillfully weaves real patient stories with clinical expertise, offering a practical and accessible resource for individuals grappling with restless legs syndrome (RLS) and their supportive partners and caregivers. Delving into diagnosis, treatment options, and the delicate balance of medication, this book not only educates but creates an empathetic connection, inviting readers to feel as if they are in Dr. Spector's office, navigating the complexities of RLS together. This will be a go-to resource for both providers and patients who are tackling RLS."

—**Charlene Gamaldo**, MD, Professor, Neurology, Medical Director,
JH Center for Sleep and Wellness

"Finally, a source of scientific knowledge, sage guidance, and empowering advice. If you have restless legs, as I do, the information in this well-written book will calm your legs and your mind. A must-buy."

—**Samantha Shad**, RLS Patient

"I have sought treatment for RLS over the past 10 years and Dr. Spector has validated many of my experiences and struggles with this condition; that in itself provides an important degree of relief. Dr. Spector's plain language explanation interspersed with personal stories from RLS patients make this book a valuable resource for RLS patients and RLS families, as well as healthcare professionals seeking to understand the condition and its human impacts."

—**Kathy Kinkema**, RLS Patient

David C. Spencer, MD, FAAN
Editor, *Brain & Life* Books®
Professor of Neurology
Oregon Health and Science University
Portland, OR

Other Titles in the *Brain & Life*® Books Series

Navigating Life with a Brain Tumor
Lynne P. Taylor, MD, FAAN; Alyx B. Porter Umphrey, MD; and
Diane Richard

Navigating the Complexities of Stroke
Louis R. Caplan, MD, FAAN

Navigating Life with Multiple Sclerosis
Kathleen Costello, MS, ANP-BC, MSCN; Ben W. Thrower, MD; and
Barbara S. Giesser, MD

Navigating Life with Epilepsy
David C. Spencer, MD, FAAN

Navigating Life with Amyotrophic Lateral Sclerosis
Mark B. Bromberg, MD, PhD, FAAN, and Diane Banks Bromberg, JD

Navigating Life with Migraine and Other Headaches
William B. Young, MD, FAAN, FANA, FAHS, and Stephen D. Silberstein, MD,
FAHS, FAAN, FACP

Navigating Life with Chronic Pain
Robert A. Lavin, MD, MS; Sara Clayton, PhD; and Lindsay Zilliox, MD

Navigating Life with Parkinson's Disease, Second Edition
Sotirios A. Parashos, MD, and Rose Wichmann, PT

Navigating Life with Dementia
James M. Noble, MD, MS, CPH, FAAN

Navigating the Challenges of Concussion
Michael S. Jaffee, MD, FAAN, FANA; Donna K. Broshek, PhD, ABPP-CN; and
Adrian M. Svingos, PhD

Navigating Life with Restless Legs Syndrome

Andrew R. Spector, MD, FAASM, FAAN

Associate Professor
Department of Neurology
Duke University School of Medicine
Durham, NC

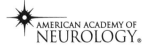

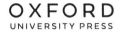

Oxford University Press is a department of the University of Oxford. It furthers
the University's objective of excellence in research, scholarship, and education
by publishing worldwide. Oxford is a registered trade mark of Oxford University
Press in the UK and certain other countries.

Published in the United States of America by Oxford University Press
198 Madison Avenue, New York, NY 10016, United States of America.

Library of Congress Cataloging-in-Publication Data
Names: Spector, Andrew R., author.
Title: Navigating life with restless legs syndrome / Andrew R. Spector.
Description: New York, NY : Oxford University Press, [2024] |
Series: Brain & life books |
Includes bibliographical references and index.
Identifiers: LCCN 2024006255 (print) | LCCN 2024006256 (ebook) |
ISBN 9780197657003 (paperback) | ISBN 9780197657027 (epub) |
ISBN 9780197657034 (ebook)
Subjects: LCSH: Restless legs syndrome—Popular works. |
Restless legs syndrome—Treatment—Popular works.
Classification: LCC RC548.5.S64 2024 (print) | LCC RC548.5 (ebook) |
DDC 616.8/498—dc23/eng/20240227
LC record available at https://lccn.loc.gov/2024006255
LC ebook record available at https://lccn.loc.gov/2024006256

DOI: 10.1093/oso/9780197657003.001.0001

This material is not intended to be, and should not be considered, a substitute for medical
or other professional advice. Treatment for the conditions described in this material is
highly dependent on the individual circumstances. And, while this material is designed
to offer accurate information with respect to the subject matter covered and to be current
as of the time it was written, research and knowledge about medical and health issues
is constantly evolving and dose schedules for medications are being revised continually,
with new side effects recognized and accounted for regularly. Readers must therefore
always check the product information and clinical procedures with the most up-to-date
published product information and data sheets provided by the manufacturers and the
most recent codes of conduct and safety regulation. The publisher and the authors make
no representations or warranties to readers, express or implied, as to the accuracy or
completeness of this material. Without limiting the foregoing, the publisher and the authors
make no representations or warranties as to the accuracy or efficacy of the drug dosages
mentioned in the material. The authors and the publisher do not accept, and expressly
disclaim, any responsibility for any liability, loss, or risk that may be claimed or incurred as
a consequence of the use and/or application of any of the contents of this material.

Printed by Sheridan Books, Inc., United States of America

This book is dedicated to my patients past, present, and future who have taught me more about restless legs syndrome than any book or journal ever could. RLS is treatable. You need not suffer forever.

CONTENTS

About the *Brain & Life®* Books Series | ix
Preface | xi

1. What is RLS? | 1

2. Why Me? | 15

3. What Causes RLS? | 29

4. Consequences of RLS | 37

5. Iron Therapy | 55

6. Treatment of RLS Without Prescription Drugs | 71

7. Dopamine Agonists for RLS | 85

8. Gabapentinoids for RLS | 99

9. Opioids for RLS | 111

10. Benzodiazepines for RLS | 127

11. Additional Medications for RLS | 135

12. RLS in Pregnancy | 147

13. RLS with Other Illnesses | 155

14. Periodic Limb Movements | 171

15. RLS in Vulnerable Populations | 177

16. Information for Loved Ones and Caregivers | 187

17. Unanswered Questions and the Future of
    RLS Management | 201

ACKNOWLEDGMENTS | 211
TREATMENT ALGORITHM | 215
GLOSSARY | 217
RESOURCES AND FURTHER READING | 235
ABOUT *BRAIN & LIFE* AND THE AMERICAN ACADEMY
  OF NEUROLOGY | 237
INDEX | 239

ABOUT THE *BRAIN & LIFE*®
BOOKS SERIES

What was the first thing you thought when you learned you or a family member had a neurologic condition? Perhaps you were confused, uncertain, afraid, or maybe even in denial. A common thread is often the realization that life has changed and may continue to change, but also uncertainty about exactly what that means or what to expect. And yet, neurologic conditions themselves inevitably change—sometimes quickly, in a matter of seconds or minutes, and sometimes gradually over months or even years.

With any new diagnosis—especially one that is potentially life changing—you may not be prepared to take in and process large amounts of new information on the spot. And even under the best circumstances, each condition comes with the need to learn a new language and understand the necessary tests, underlying causes, and right treatments. It may be difficult to wrap your arms around a great deal of information in what are often time-limited appointments with your neurologist. Understanding your new diagnosis and how to manage it is a gradual process, and you will inevitably have questions with the passage of time and reflection. Learning about your condition can help you understand what the most useful and accurate information is to share with your neurology team, allowing you to fully participate in treatment decisions.

But facts and information are only part of the picture. You may have questions about how to manage your day-to-day life with a neurologic condition: whether in terms of your career, your home, your relationships, or, in some instances, long-term planning and care. We designed the *Brain & Life* Books series to help you address some of the fears, concerns, and difficult emotions you may feel, such as grief and worry, by harnessing the power of accurate and timely information to help guide you and your family through the change brought about by a neurologic diagnosis. The books share stories of others who have traveled down paths like the one you are on to reinforce the fact that you are not alone.

We selected the authors of the series carefully with these goals in mind. First and foremost, all authors are respected experts in their field, and the information in the *Brain & Life* Books series is accurate, up-to-date, and written to be understandable to someone with no medical background. Experts from the premier neurology organization in the world, the American Academy of Neurology, and the oldest and largest university press in the world, Oxford University Press, carefully review each book to ensure the highest quality. But we also chose our authors because of their experience and ability to connect with patients and their families. The experiences and feelings you are having now have been dealt with and managed successfully by our authors and their patients. Our authors will share with you best practices, stories, and pearls of advice that will leave you with a feeling that your diagnosis is manageable— you can do this. We have highlighted all key terms when first used that you and your family should know, and we have included them in a comprehensive glossary at the back of the book.

The *Brain & Life* Books series was written with you in mind, whether you have been diagnosed yourself or are a family member, caregiver, or friend of someone who has been, as a resource for successfully navigating life with a neurologic condition.

David Spencer, MD, FAAN

Editor, *Brain & Life* Books®

Professor of Neurology

Oregon Health and Science University, Portland, OR

PREFACE

Do you find your legs begin to have unpleasant sensations when you sit still later in the day or when you go to bed? Does this discomfort improve if you get up and move? Then you probably have restless legs syndrome. It's also known as restless "leg" syndrome or Willis-Ekbom disease, but you might have your own name for it. One website has recorded 120 different names that people living with restless legs syndrome have come up with for their own symptoms. My favorites are "the wheeby geebees" and "the creepers." In this book, we'll call it RLS. Whatever you call it, if you're living with it, you know it's no joke.

I developed a passion for treating RLS after seeing so many patients suffering with this condition over my more than 10 years in practice as a sleep medicine physician. Patients have told me that having RLS is worse than undergoing chemotherapy for cancer and that they're considering cutting off their legs or committing suicide because they can't tolerate it anymore (true stories), so I know how big of a problem RLS is.

Unfortunately, I continue to hear comments like "No doctor ever took these symptoms seriously before" and "I didn't know there was anything that could be done about it." I take RLS very seriously, and there's definitely something that can be done about it. My goal is to empower you, the reader with RLS, and your loved ones with knowledge about RLS and how we treat it so that you can work with your health care providers to start feeling—and sleeping—better.

While many medical conditions get long and confusing names that only make sense to neurologists and speakers of Latin, and others get named after people you've probably never heard of (like Parkinson's disease), RLS, thankfully, is very aptly named to explain what is actually happening. Usually. For most people with RLS, RLS means having a restlessness in their legs. Some people, though, get RLS in their arms, backs, or even genitals. For simplicity, I will refer to all of these variants as "RLS."

If you are experiencing these unpleasant symptoms, then this book is for you. And if you are a spouse, partner, family member, or caregiver of someone with RLS, Chapter 16 in particular is for you. I will attempt to give you all the information you ever wanted to know about RLS and maybe some information you didn't even know you wanted. We will cover RLS basics, like how we make the diagnosis (Chapter 1), and then move on to discussing who is at risk for getting RLS and what might trigger it (Chapter 2). We will also cover some basic neuroscience that will help you understand where RLS comes from (Chapter 3). I promise not to get too science-y, but I do want you to have a sense of why your brain is doing this to you, and what the impact might be on your body (Chapter 4).

After we cover those foundational principles, we'll move on to treatments (Chapters 5 to 11). We'll spend a lot of time on this subject because this is probably what you're most interested in. Prescription drugs, nonprescription drugs, nondrug prescriptions, home remedies, and experimental therapies will all be reviewed. We will also cover RLS in specific populations, such as pregnant women and older adults (Chapters 12 to 14). Although children can suffer from RLS, this book is directed to adults.

RLS is treated in a variety of health care settings, such as primary care clinics, general neurology clinics, and sleep medicine clinics, to name a few. In these settings, patients will encounter physicians, nurse practitioners, physician assistants, and possibly even more kinds of health care providers. In this book, the term "provider" will cover the range of possible health care professionals who care for patients with RLS. In case vignettes throughout the book, one type of provider might be used as an example, but in these cases, there is no specific importance to which category of provider is mentioned. Quality health care can be delivered in all these settings by all these types of providers.

I hope you find this book informative, helpful, and even a little entertaining. Throughout the book, there are stories of patients— some who are real (with their permission and their names changed) and some who are composites—that represent common themes from many patients. You will probably identify with many of these stories, and I am optimistic that they will give you hope as you see others like you getting relief from this maddening condition.

Before we begin, we must acknowledge the irony that one of the hardest things for a person with RLS to do is to sit still for a long period of time to read a book. Thankfully, there's no rush. This book isn't going anywhere. Take frequent breaks to walk around. Try reading earlier in the day before the symptoms hit you. Or if you are on medications for RLS and they don't sedate you too much, try taking some before sitting down to read in the evening. We'll get through this together.

CHAPTER 1

What is RLS?

In this chapter, you will learn:

- What the term "restless legs syndrome" means
- What are the classic features of restless legs syndrome
- How restless legs syndrome is diagnosed
- How restless legs syndrome differs from other conditions that affect the legs
- When you should seek help for your restless legs syndrome

Introduction

Restless legs syndrome, also known as RLS, is one of the most under-appreciated conditions in neurology. It might not be fatal, but it sure can make you miserable. It can completely destroy your quality of life. For some people, that means they can't enjoy a movie or a play because sitting in a theater for 2 hours would be insufferable. For others, traveling in a car, especially as a passenger, or on an airplane, where leg room is limited, can bring untold distress. Many people with RLS are unable to put their legs up and enjoy some television at the end of the day. And if these problems weren't bad enough, when RLS prevents you from sleeping, the nighttime frustration and daytime exhaustion can become unbearable.

This chapter will give you a broad overview of what RLS is and what it is not. We will cover the typical RLS symptoms along with the criteria used to diagnose it. There are many other diagnoses that cause leg symptoms, and the information in this chapter will help you differentiate RLS from the conditions that mimic it. If all this information gets overwhelming, remember, you aren't responsible for diagnosing yourself. Talk to your health care providers about your symptoms and let them help you sort it all out.

> Sandy is a 67-year-old woman who complains every night to her husband that her legs are bothering her. Every evening, she gets a creepy-crawly feeling in her legs that makes her get up and move. She asks her husband to rub her legs for her, and he obliges. If he's not there, she is up, pacing around the house. Her husband persuades her to see her doctor because "this can't be normal," he says. Sandy's doctor quickly recognizes her condition and diagnoses her with RLS. Sandy hasn't heard of this before and asks for more information.

Restless legs syndrome is a **sensorimotor disorder** in which people experience an unpleasant urge to move, often in the legs, that is worse later in the day and better with movement. We use the word "restless" because that's what many patients describe, but there are a variety of different sensations that would still qualify for an RLS diagnosis. Patients may describe the feeling that ants are crawling on their skin or that they have a deep itching or gnawing sensation in their bones. There are many possibilities for how you might experience RLS, but the sensations are universally unpleasant. The medical word for these abnormal sensations is "**dysesthesia**." In this book, I'll often use the word "restless" as a stand-in for all the different symptoms that one might experience with RLS.

Pain is not a classic feature of RLS, but there is a painful form that some patients may experience. The most common types of pain are described as burning sensations or dull aches. While the painful form of RLS is much less common, the existence of a painful form can make the diagnosis trickier because these patients don't fit the traditional description of RLS symptoms.

Just as "restless" doesn't account for the whole spectrum of sensations, "legs" doesn't account for the different places in the body that you might experience symptoms. While RLS is most frequently experienced in both legs, it can affect just one leg, or it could affect the arms, the torso, or the genitals. There are even reports of restless anus syndrome. We currently have no explanation for why RLS shows up in different places in different people.

The final word in the name is "**syndrome**." A syndrome is essentially a collection of symptoms that exist together. In medicine, we usually use the word "syndrome" when there isn't a clearly understood cause for the symptoms. The word "disease" is more commonly used when there is a specific, known cause. With recent research advancing what is known about the causes of RLS, one might argue that we have reached the stage where we could call it a disease, but the term "RLS" is so engrained now that it's unlikely to change anytime soon. That being said, "syndrome" is still appropriate as there are almost certainly different causes of these symptoms in different people, which would mean RLS is not a singular disease.

There was an effort to change the name recently to **Willis-Ekbom disease (WED)**, so you'll see this on a lot of medical websites, but this name has never really gained popular usage. For what it's worth, Dr. Willis was a British physician who described the condition in the 1680s, and Dr. Ekbom, a Swedish neurologist, did so in the 1940s. Personally, as the name RLS is more descriptive, even if not entirely accurate, I prefer it over WED.

THE DIAGNOSIS

Now that we've explored the name, let's talk about how providers figure out if you have it. One of the unique features of RLS is that if you think you have it, you probably do. You don't need to undergo any testing for a provider to make the diagnosis. There are four key questions your provider will ask if you are suspected of having RLS.

1. Do you have a restless or unpleasant sensation in your legs (or elsewhere)?
2. Does the unpleasant sensation worsen later in the day, typically in the evening or nighttime?
3. Does the unpleasant sensation worsen when you're resting or holding still?
4. Does the unpleasant sensation improve if you get up and move around?

If you answer yes to these four questions, you meet the basic criteria for a diagnosis of RLS. I've seen patients who I am certain have RLS who do not answer yes to all four, but the official definition of RLS requires four yeses. There is also a caveat that your symptoms aren't better explained by another diagnosis; conditions that mimic RLS are discussed later in this chapter.

RLS is considered a "**clinical diagnosis.**" This means that once we suspect RLS, we do not need to confirm it with a test. That said, there have been attempts to measure RLS objectively. There is a test for RLS, called the **suggested immobilization test**, abbreviated as SIT (clever, right?), but this is not regularly used in practice and is not included in the guidelines for diagnosing RLS. It can be used in research, for example, to measure changes in leg movements after administering a treatment.

A SIT requires you to sit still with outstretched legs for 60 minutes at 9:00 PM to quantify the frequency of involuntary leg jerks that occur while you rate the severity of your restlessness. Realistically, most patients with RLS can describe exactly what would happen if they attempted to do this, making the formal test unnecessary. Formal sleep testing, officially called polysomnography (PSG) and colloquially referred to as a **sleep study**, is also not needed for the diagnosis of RLS. More than that, a diagnosis of RLS cannot be made from a PSG, although this is a common misperception.

> Rajesh is a 35-year-old man who went to see his primary care doctor to request an evaluation for loud snoring that was bothering his roommate. His doctor was concerned that Rajesh had *obstructive sleep apnea (OSA)* and ordered a sleep study. She also scheduled him for an appointment in a sleep medicine clinic to follow up on the results of the sleep study. A week later, she called Rajesh to let him know that his study results showed that he had both OSA and RLS, and that he should follow up with the sleep medicine clinic for treatment of both.

RLS versus PLMS

At Rajesh's sleep medicine appointment, he told the **physician assistant** (PA) that he was there for OSA and RLS. The PA talked to him about OSA and then asked him how often he is bothered by his legs feeling restless at night. Rajesh responded that his legs never bother him at night, and the only reason he had brought it up was because his primary doctor told him that he had been diagnosed with RLS during his sleep study. The PA reassured Rajesh that despite what he'd been told, he does not have RLS because he doesn't have any bothersome leg symptoms.

If—like Rajesh—you were told that your sleep study showed RLS, you're not alone; it's an unfortunately common error. While sleep studies might contain clues about RLS, your symptoms are what matter, not what shows up on a sleep study.

The PA explained to Rajesh that he had **periodic limb movements of sleep,** or **PLMS**, which are not the same as RLS. PLMS, or the closely related but less common condition **periodic limb movements of wake**, are leg jerks that occur at a semiregular frequency. If you have had a sleep study, you will see these recorded on the report. In addition, the report will indicate a **periodic limb movement index**, which is the frequency at which these events occur. While RLS and PLMS frequently occur in the same people, you can have one and not the other.

The key difference is in the sensations you experience. RLS is highly unpleasant and occurs when you are awake, whereas PLMS can be completely unrecognized by the person who has them and—as the name indicates—occur during sleep. It is often the bedpartner of someone with PLMS who is most bothered by the movements.

Periodic limb movements of wake are spontaneous leg jerks that occur prior to falling asleep but not associated with the restlessness that characterizes RLS. If you have both the restlessness and the jerks, the diagnosis is RLS; there's no need for a second diagnosis of periodic limb movements of wake. A comprehensive discussion of PLMS can be found in Chapter 14.

It's possible for PLMS to become so frequent that they disrupt sleep enough to cause daytime symptoms. In that case we call it **periodic limb movement disorder (PLMD)**. PLMD is a challenging diagnosis to make, though, as it can be very difficult to determine when the PLMS are sufficiently disruptive to call them a disorder, particularly when other sleep problems, like obstructive sleep apnea, are also present.

The typical strategy with PLMS is to treat everything else first, and if you still aren't feeling better, then a reasonable next step would be to treat the limb movements. Contrast this to RLS, where patients are able to tell us exactly how disruptive their restlessness is. Treatment for RLS is initiated when you decide you need treatment. While this book is about RLS and not PLMD, the treatment strategies for RLS are essentially the same as what is used to treat PLMD.

The bottom line here is that RLS and PLMS are not the same phenomenon. If you have PLMS on your sleep studies but no symptoms of RLS, then you probably don't require treatment. And if you are treated, it should be because you have PLMD (i.e., PLMS that disrupt your sleep enough to cause daytime symptoms). If treatment of PLMD does not lead to an improvement in symptoms, then treatment should be stopped. There is no known value in treating most people who happen to show PLMS on their sleep studies, particularly those with no other symptoms.

Conditions that MIMIC RLS

Although the diagnostic criteria for RLS seem straightforward, one of the classic teachings in medicine is "patients don't read textbooks," which means not everyone with RLS will report the same symptoms or behave the same way. Sometimes, conditions that aren't RLS have symptoms that are similar to RLS, making the diagnosis less clear. In this section, we'll review conditions that can be mistaken for RLS and how you and your provider can distinguish between them.

RLS versus NEUROPATHY

The trick in making an RLS diagnosis is figuring out if there is a better explanation for the symptoms. There are conditions that mimic RLS, so part of your provider's job is to sort this out with you. What makes this even more confusing is that you might have more than one problem. For example, some people have **peripheral neuropathy**, which means chronic **nerve** damage, usually in the feet and lower legs.

Peripheral neuropathy also causes uncomfortable sensations in the legs, so it can be a challenge for providers to figure out if your symptoms are from neuropathy or RLS. And since people with neuropathy are more likely to have RLS than people without neuropathy, we often see both conditions together. It's important to work with your provider to determine if you have RLS, neuropathy, or both.

> George is an 80-year-old man with a history of diabetes who is seeing his primary care doctor for unpleasant sensations in his feet. He tells his doctor that it feels like a burning pain, just in his feet. It's worse at night when he's trying to sleep, but it's there all day. He hasn't noticed that it gets any better when he's moving compared to when he's sitting or lying down. He also doesn't think he can feel his feet as well anymore, yet they always seem cold to him.

George's doctor's job is to figure out what is causing George to have these sensations. When George reported uncomfortable feelings that got worse at night, George's doctor considered RLS as the cause, but there were too many other elements in George's story that led his doctor in another direction. Did you catch them? His feet felt like they were burning or cold (unusual sensations for RLS), the pain was there all day (not just at night) and he felt no better when he was moving (a requirement for an RLS diagnosis). This is not likely to be RLS.

While none of them is perfect, there are some general guidelines to help differentiate neuropathy from RLS. First, neuropathy tends to cause more pain than RLS. As we talked about earlier in this chapter, there is a painful form of RLS, but since most RLS is not painful, the presence of pain usually suggests an underlying neuropathy.

Second, neuropathy symptoms tend to be present throughout the day, while RLS is more likely to be present only in the evening or nighttime. Neuropathy pain might be worse at night, but it tends to have less of a daily cycle than RLS does.

Finally, numbness is a symptom that is only present in neuropathy. If you have numbness, such as difficulty perceiving temperature changes, this is a sign that you should be evaluated for neuropathy.

Since diabetes is one of the major causes of neuropathy, all patients with diabetes need to be evaluated for neuropathy during a workup for RLS.

A brief overview of neuropathy

A full discussion of neuropathy is beyond the scope of this book, but given the overlap between RLS and neuropathy, it's important to understand some neuropathy basics. Neuropathies can be categorized in many ways, but one of them is whether there is damage to the **large-** or **small-fiber nerves**. **Large-fiber neuropathy** is a disease of the nerves that controls strength and the sensations of light touch, pressure, and vibration. **Small-fiber neuropathy**, by comparison, affects the sensations of pain and temperature, and can also affect the way the body controls **unconscious** (also known as **autonomic**) functions, such as heart rate and blood pressure regulation, sweating, and digestion.

Peripheral neuropathy can refer to damage to the large fibers, small fibers, or both. Often, a thorough physical examination can give your provider a sense of which nerve fibers are affected. Additional testing frequently includes a **nerve conduction study**, which is typically done in conjunction with an **electromyogram (EMG)**. These are electrical tests on the nerves and muscles. Nerve conduction studies can tell you if you have a large-fiber neuropathy, but they cannot tell you if you have a small-fiber neuropathy.

If you have a large-fiber neuropathy, there is no need to test separately for a small-fiber neuropathy because we have already confirmed the presence of neuropathy. However, if your nerve conduction study is normal, you might be recommended to undergo a **biopsy** of the skin on your leg. This skin sample can be analyzed to look for damage to small-fiber nerves under a microscope. This test is not perfect, though, and not all providers recommend them. Some providers will make the diagnosis of a small-fiber neuropathy based on your history and physical examination alone.

If you are diagnosed with neuropathy, you will then be evaluated for why you might have developed this problem, and treatment can be considered. If you do not have neuropathy, though, it is more likely that your unpleasant sensations are related to RLS.

Myoclonus

There are several other RLS mimics besides neuropathy, including **myoclonus**, which means muscle jerk. It's possible with myoclonus to have symptoms that get worse when you relax and better when you are active, which is the same pattern we see in RLS. Given that RLS makes people want to jerk their legs, it's easy to see how these two could be confused. It gets even more confusing because these conditions can respond to the same medications (see Chapter 8). The primary difference between them is that myoclonus is purely a movement problem. The jerks are not preceded by the uncomfortable feelings of RLS or the urge to move. The jerks occur suddenly and unexpectedly.

The most common example of myoclonus affecting sleep is **hypnic jerks**, also known as **sleep-onset myoclonus**. Many, if not most, people have experienced the sensation at least once in their lives where they are just about to fall asleep and the body suddenly jerks them back awake. Sometimes this feels like you're falling before the body suddenly stiffens up. It is usually straightforward to differentiate hypnic jerks from RLS as hypnic jerks only occur at the transition from wake to sleep, but muscle jerks that occur earlier in the evening when relaxing can be more difficult to distinguish from RLS. And just like with neuropathy, it's possible to have RLS and myoclonus at the same time.

Maria is a 70-year-old woman who is seeking help from a sleep doctor for leg problems. She says that she gets into bed at night and starts jerking so much that she can't fall asleep. This has been going on for several years, and it's making her miserable and sleep deprived. She was prescribed medication for RLS, but it hasn't stopped the movements. Her sleep doctor added a different medication to reduce the muscle jerks, which helped her sleep.

Maria presented a challenge for her sleep doctor because the initial symptoms sounded like RLS, but she didn't respond to RLS medications as her doctor had expected. Her doctor then considered myoclonus as the primary problem and started treatment for that instead. In Maria's case, her doctor weaned her off the RLS medication once the myoclonus was treated, at which point Maria had classic RLS symptoms again. She had both diagnoses, which was only made clear by her response to treatment. It was only when taking both medications that she slept well.

RLS versus nighttime leg cramps

Nighttime leg cramps are also different from RLS. Leg cramps can be horribly painful, which, as we've discussed, is not typical of RLS. They often come out of the blue, last a couple of minutes, then go away on their own. Unlucky people will have them more than once in a night, but leg cramps don't persist for hours like RLS can. A cramp is a specific event, even if cramps recur over and over for hours.

Leg cramps are more likely to wake people up out of sleep than RLS. If you're having frequent leg cramps, it's important to speak to your provider to try to figure out why. If there is a cause, like a medication side effect or abnormal calcium levels in the blood, for example, the leg cramps will get better by correcting these problems. Otherwise, there are unfortunately very few effective treatments for leg cramps.

RLS versus drug-induced akathisia

The constant movement and fidgeting that occurs in RLS goes by the medical term **akathisia**. Akathisia is an inability to sit still. Other than RLS, akathisia can be associated with **psychiatric** medications, such as **antipsychotics** or, less commonly, **antidepressants** (Table 1.1). It is therefore not surprising that these medications are

TABLE 1.1 **Examples of medications that can cause akathisia**

Drug name	Drug class
Chlorpromazine	Antipsychotic
Citalopram	Antidepressant
Fluoxetine	Antidepressant
Haloperidol	Antipsychotic
Paroxetine	Antidepressant
Prochlorperazine	Antinausea
Promethazine	Antinausea

known to exacerbate RLS, but they can also cause akathisia in patients who do not have underlying RLS.

Medication-induced akathisia does not have the daily rhythm of RLS, which affects people predominantly in the evenings and nights. RLS patients will nearly always be able to sit still long enough to be able to complete an office visit, but patients with akathisia will often fidget throughout the appointment. People with akathisia may do better when given an **antihistamine** such as diphenhydramine, while people with RLS tend to get worse.

RLS versus painful legs moving toes syndrome

A rare condition that can mimic RLS is called **painful legs moving toes syndrome**. Yes, that's a real name of a real diagnosis. This condition can be differentiated from RLS because the movements tend to be unconscious, writhing movements in the toes rather than whole leg movements that are under more conscious control in RLS. The pain in painful legs moving toes syndrome is in the lower leg, while the abnormal sensations in RLS can be in the upper or lower leg or both. Painful legs moving toes syndrome is also not specifically an evening and nighttime phenomenon, so if these symptoms are most severe in the morning or occur throughout the day, it's less likely to be RLS.

Confirming your RLS diagnosis

At this point, if you are still wondering if you have RLS and not one of the other disorders that appear like RLS, please see your provider for an evaluation or to get a referral to a specialist for an evaluation. Inaccurate diagnoses can lead to incorrect treatments with possibly harmful side effects. Some readers likely already have formal diagnoses by physicians, while other readers have diagnosed themselves.

To the self-diagnosed group, you might be wondering if it's even necessary to see a health care provider about this problem. That decision should be based on the severity of your symptoms. If you are suffering, then yes, you should definitely seek help. There's no need to suffer for a condition that can be effectively treated. But if your symptoms are mild and you would not want any treatments, there is nothing dangerous about delaying medical care for RLS. Unlike cancer screening tests, this is not a case of early detection saving lives. Essentially, the time to seek help is when you don't want to live with the discomfort anymore.

Most of the time, diagnosing RLS is relatively straightforward. The symptoms are often classic: an uncomfortable sensation, often an urge to move, that is worse at night, worse at rest, and better with movement. However, human bodies have a way of doing things that don't always fit the textbook definitions of diseases, and sometimes more than one problem is going on at the same time. This can make diagnosing RLS more challenging. Your health care team can help you determine if you have RLS.

The coming chapters will explore who is most at risk for RLS and what common triggers can make it worse. Then, we'll dive a little deeper into the science behind RLS and its causes.

CHAPTER 2

Why Me?

In this chapter, you will learn:

- How common is RLS
- Which ages, genders, and races are most likely to have RLS
- What medical conditions are often seen alongside RLS
- How to interpret iron tests in the setting of RLS
- What medications and substances can trigger RLS

Introduction

As far as we know, there is no one on Earth who is immune to RLS. It can happen to anyone, but some people are more at risk than others. This chapter will review the various factors that place people at risk for RLS. You might have one or more than one of these conditions, or you might have none. Not everyone with RLS can identify a clear reason why they have it. While a few of these risk factors are at least somewhat under your control, others—like your age—are not.

One common contributing factor to RLS is low iron, and this chapter will explain how to understand iron test results, because it's not as simple as the lab reports make it seem. It's also important for you to know if something you're taking, such as a prescription medication, could be making your RLS worse. This chapter will give you information on what might be triggering your RLS.

Across the world, RLS seems to occur in anywhere from 1% to 14% of people. This large range is a result of different research strategies. Who is studied and how they are studied can affect the results. For instance, asking someone if they have ever had symptoms in their lives and asking if those symptoms occur every day will yield different answers. Even if we use an estimate on the low end of the range, a condition that affects 3% of the population is still very common. That means that there are probably at least 10 million Americans with RLS.

As with many conditions in medicine, there are differences in the frequency of RLS associated with age, sex, and race. While children and young adults can develop RLS, the risk of RLS is higher in middle and older age groups (i.e., over age 40). Another risk factor for RLS is being born female. Study after study has shown that females are more likely to suffer from RLS than males, possibly up to twice as likely. Nevertheless, there are still millions of males out there with RLS, so the fact that females are more likely to get RLS should not dissuade males from getting evaluated or treated for it.

Likewise, using the racial categorizations of the United States, most studies have found that White people are more likely than Black people to have RLS, but that doesn't mean that Black people don't get RLS, just that it is less common. It also seems that RLS is less common in people of Asian ancestry based on studies both in the United States and in several Asian countries, but even at a relatively lower rate of 1%, that means many millions of Asians suffer from RLS. As a result, it's best not to focus on age, sex, or race to help with the diagnosis of RLS. It is such a universal condition that it's still common even among groups for which it is *relatively* rare.

It is more important to focus on the health conditions—instead of the demographics—that place people at higher risk for RLS. One of these conditions, pregnancy, will be covered in depth in Chapter 12, so it will not be addressed here. Other conditions associated with having a higher risk of RLS include stroke, **iron deficiency**, peripheral neuropathy (see Chapter 1), **kidney disease, heart** failure, **multiple sclerosis**, and **vitamin D deficiency**. While not an exhaustive list, these are common conditions that have a strong association with RLS.

> Ernest is an 85-year-old man who had a *stroke* 3 months ago and is seeing his *neurologist* for a follow-up visit. He tells his neurologist that since his stroke he's had restlessness in his legs that makes it uncomfortable for him to sit in his favorite recliner at night. This is particularly bothersome because he has not been able to walk independently since his stroke, so he can't get up and move, which is the only thing that helps his legs feel better. His neurologist diagnoses him with RLS and explains that he is at risk for this condition due to his age and his history of stroke.

Iron deficiency

Iron deficiency—specifically *brain* **iron deficiency**—is a common cause of RLS. The importance of iron to both the cause and treatment of RLS can't be overstated, but iron levels are tricky. The amount of iron in the brain can be too low even if the levels of iron in your blood are considered "normal." Blood counts are not related to the iron levels in the brain, and you cannot rely on them as a proxy for brain iron levels. The only way to find out exactly how much iron is in your brain is to do a **spinal tap** and check the levels of iron in the spinal fluid, but to the relief of many patients, this isn't something that is done in routine, clinical practice.

Thankfully, some brave volunteers underwent spinal tap testing already, and we now know that people with RLS have lower levels of brain iron on average than those without RLS. Some groups, mostly outside the United States, are doing ultrasounds of the brain to look for signs of iron deficiency that way, but this is not yet being done even in specialty clinics in the United States. The key point to remember is that just because the lab says your iron level is normal doesn't mean you have enough iron in your brain.

To be precise, when talking about lab tests for iron levels, I'm referring to two in particular: **ferritin** and **transferrin saturation**. Ferritin is a **blood protein** that stores iron. Even though you might see a test result labeled "iron" on your blood work, the ferritin level is a more reliable way to assess your body's iron. If you are getting iron levels checked, it's likely that your ferritin level is actually what is being reviewed by your provider.

Food and the time of day your blood is drawn both affect the ferritin results, so your blood draw should occur first thing in the morning before breakfast. You also should not take iron pills or eat a high-iron meal (e.g., beef) before getting your blood iron levels assessed. One patient of mine registered a transferrin saturation of 81% (extremely high) after having taken an iron pill in the morning and 19% (mildly low) when the level was rechecked after not taking the pill. Her iron levels did not naturally drop that much between the two tests; the first one was falsely elevated due to the pill itself. Make sure there are at least 12 hours, but preferably 24 hours, between taking the pill and having your blood drawn.

Interpreting ferritin levels can be tricky because the results can be high for reasons other than having high iron. Inflammation from conditions such as infections, **autoimmune diseases**, cancer, and kidney disease could make the ferritin level go up even if you have low iron. That's why it's important to also check your transferrin saturation.

Transferrin is a protein that binds to iron in the blood, and we can measure how much of it is bound to the iron in your blood. If your body has too little iron, most of the transferrin will not have iron bound to it, which we refer to as a low saturation. This is another indication of iron deficiency. If either the ferritin or the transferrin saturation percentage is low, you might be iron deficient. In the context of

RLS, transferrin saturations below 20% are considered low, with 20% to 25% being borderline low.

Laboratories will report that ferritin levels as low as 11 or 12 μg/L (micrograms per liter) are "normal." In the RLS world, though, this is severely iron deficient, as blood iron levels this low can nearly guarantee that brain iron is very low. Current guidelines for the treatment of RLS say that ferritin should be at least 75 μg/L, as it takes at least that much blood iron to have sufficient brain iron in people with RLS. Even that amount might be too low for many people, and some RLS experts suggest this should be at least 100 μg/L. One common rule of thumb is that the ferritin level should be higher than your age because ferritin levels naturally go up as we age, so if you're older than 75, your ferritin target is even higher than 75. There's a lot of room between 11 and 75 for people with RLS to be told (improperly) that their iron levels are fine when they most certainly aren't. This is one of the most common errors in RLS management.

Anyone with RLS and a ferritin less than 75 μg/L should be treated with iron therapy unless doing so would negatively impact any other health conditions a patient may have, though this would be rare. There will be much more on iron therapy in Chapter 5. Figure 2.1 provides an algorithm for interpreting iron tests. Interpreting iron testing is complicated, and your provider will help you sort all of this out.

The reason iron in the blood and the brain are different is because iron doesn't move from the blood into the brain very easily due to the **blood-brain barrier** (Figure 2.2). The blood-brain barrier is a great system of interlocking cells that protect the brain from anything circulating in the blood that would be harmful to it. In the case of iron, though, it can make it hard for your brain to get enough. Your body must transfer iron from the blood across the blood-brain barrier, and patients with RLS don't seem able to do this very efficiently. Scientists have even found that this inefficiency to transport iron across the blood-brain barrier has a **genetic** component that can pass from parent to child. Due to this difficulty

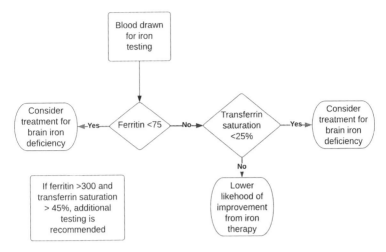

FIGURE 2.1 Algorithm for understanding iron test results in the context of RLS.

transporting the iron, you can have a normal amount of blood iron and still have low brain iron.

Makena is a 52-year-old female who made an appointment at the local sleep clinic for help managing her RLS. She was referred by her primary care provider. The sleep doctor asked Makena if she's ever had her iron levels checked. Makena responded that her primary care provider told her that her blood counts were normal, so she did not need iron testing. The sleep doctor explained to Makena that many people with RLS have iron deficiency with normal blood counts. The doctor ordered lab testing for Makena, which revealed low iron. After discussing the pros and cons, the sleep doctor ordered an intravenous (IV) infusion of iron. The doctor told Makena that about 6 to 8 weeks after her infusion, she should start to feel better. Makena received the infusion, and when she returned to sleep clinic 3 months after the initial visit, her RLS was much improved.

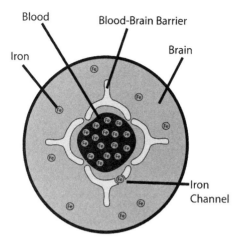

Blood

Blood-Brain Barrier

Iron

Brain

Iron
Channel

FIGURE 2.2 Diagram of the blood-brain barrier. Fe represents iron, and even though there is a high concentration of iron in the blood (dark gray), there is not as much in the brain (light gray). This is due to the brain cells ("blood-brain barrier") that form a barrier between the blood and the brain. Note the channel (bottom right) that allows only a small amount of iron into the brain at a time. (Figure credit: Adaora Spector)

Contributing health conditions

Moving beyond brain iron deficiency, another very common association with RLS is peripheral neuropathy. Chapter 1 discussed how to decide if the discomfort in your legs is due to RLS or peripheral neuropathy, but they often co-occur, and the peripheral neuropathy can worsen symptoms of RLS. It's possible that people who have both neuropathy and RLS have somewhat different symptoms, such as more pain. Thankfully, there is overlap between the treatments for the symptoms of neuropathy and for RLS (see Chapter 8).

People with kidney disease, especially those who have severe kidney disease requiring **dialysis**, are also more likely than people without kidney disease to have RLS—around two to three times more likely. Whether it's the kidney disease that causes the RLS or if both diagnoses are caused by some shared underlying disease is not clear. One possibility is that toxin accumulation in the blood of a patient with kidney disease could trigger the symptoms of RLS. It's also possible that people with kidney disease are more prone to iron deficiency. A cruel irony is that people receiving dialysis must sit for long periods of time during the procedure, which can be very difficult while also suffering from RLS. RLS often improves in patients with kidney disease who receive a transplant.

Sofia is an 82-year-old female who has been a patient in a sleep clinic for the past 10 years for treatment of her RLS. She scheduled an urgent follow-up visit to discuss a rapid worsening in her symptoms. She reports that the medication she takes for her RLS is no longer helping. The sleep doctor reviews her chart and discovers that Sofia started treatment for advanced kidney failure 2 months ago. The sleep doctor discusses the role of kidney failure in RLS, adjusts her medications, and orders iron tests. The lab tests return showing iron deficiency, so the sleep doctor contacts the patient's kidney doctor to discuss getting Sofia an infusion of iron. Sofia reports back a month later to say that her symptoms, while not gone, are more tolerable now.

While kidney disease seems to be a cause of RLS, with heart disease, the relationship might go both directions. There's evidence that RLS might contribute to developing heart disease. For example, people who treat their RLS are less likely to have heart disease than people who have RLS but don't treat it. For this to apply to you, though, the RLS must be of sufficient severity to affect the quantity and quality of your sleep. It is also possible that some forms of heart disease, such as heart failure and **coronary artery disease**, contribute to the development of RLS. For example, if patients who have heart disease due to blockages in the arteries of the heart also have blockages that reduce blood flow to the legs, they might get RLS. This might be why moderate exercise, which improves blood flow to the legs, can reduce RLS symptoms.

Heart failure can also be associated with iron deficiency, which means that it could cause RLS the same way kidney failure does. The association between RLS and heart failure isn't quite as strong as it is with kidney failure. Patients with heart failure are about 1.5 times more likely than those without heart failure to have RLS.

Multiple sclerosis (MS) is another condition often associated with RLS. Nearly a third of all people with MS will also have at least some degree of RLS, and nearly one fifth of people with MS have RLS that is significant enough to disrupt their quality of life. Presumably, the changes in the brain and spinal cord that occur in MS disrupt the pathways in the brain that are responsible for RLS (see discussion of pathways in Chapter 3).

Another brain disease with a strong relationship to RLS is stroke. At the beginning of the chapter, you met Ernest, who is a good example of stroke leading to RLS. Strokes cause damage to the brain due to either a blockage in blood flow or bleeding into the brain. Most often, the symptoms of a stroke affect one side of the body, and consequently, RLS patients who have experienced a stroke may only experience RLS symptoms on one side of their body. There is also evidence that sleep disruption from severe RLS can increase the risk of stroke in the future.

One of the other causes of one-sided RLS symptoms is surgery. Patients with knee joint replacement surgery will sometimes develop RLS specifically in the leg that underwent surgery. If you have RLS prior to surgery, your legs might be generally more restless afterward, but for people who have never had RLS before they might start having symptoms on just one side. Very little research has been done on postoperative RLS, so it is not known how common it is.

Finally, for the past decade, more and more research has linked vitamin D deficiency to RLS. Patients with RLS are more likely to have vitamin D deficiency, and patients with vitamin D deficiency are more likely to have RLS. Some research has even shown improvement in RLS symptoms when vitamin D levels come up, which suggests that the low vitamin D levels were causing at least some of the RLS symptoms.

The connection to vitamin D levels is not definitive, as some research has found higher vitamin D in patients with RLS than those without RLS. Nevertheless, given that vitamin D supplementation is recommended for people with low vitamin D levels anyway, if you have RLS and low vitamin D, your provider will likely recommend you take vitamin D pills even if it doesn't help the RLS.

Medication triggers

Numerous medications, both prescription and over the counter, can exacerbate RLS. **Dopamine** is the **neurotransmitter** (a chemical messenger in the brain) that is most strongly associated with RLS. While Chapter 3 will review the science behind RLS and you'll see how dopamine is involved, in short, know that drugs that affect dopamine levels place patients at risk of developing RLS. The drugs that do this are typically **antinausea** or **antipsychotic** medications because they block dopamine transmission. See Table 2.1 for examples of medications that fall into these categories.

Mark is a 51-year-old male who has had diabetes since age 8. Over the years, he has developed several complications of his diabetes, including neuropathy and *gastroparesis*, which means his digestive system moves too slowly. He was started on a medication to help speed up his digestion, which proved helpful to relieve some of his abdominal discomfort. At his routine visit with the nurse practitioner caring for his diabetes,

(Continued)

TABLE 2.1 **Common prescription and over-the-counter medications that can exacerbate RLS**

Drug class	Common examples	Mechanism	Typical purpose(s)
Selective serotonin reuptake inhibitors (SSRI)	Fluoxetine Paroxetine Sertraline Citalopram Escitalopram	Increase serotonin	Antidepressant Antianxiety
Serotonin and norepinephrine reuptake inhibitors (SNRIs)	Duloxetine Venlafaxine	Increase serotonin and norepinephrine	Antidepressant Pain relief Menopausal hot flashes
Tricyclics/tetracyclics	Amitriptyline Nortriptyline Mirtazapine	Increase serotonin and norepinephrine	Antidepressant Induce sleep Pain relief
Dopamine antagonists	Chlorpromazine Fluphenazine Haloperidol Metoclopramide Perphenazine Prochlorperazine Promethazine Thioridazine	Block dopamine	Antinausea Antipsychotic
Antihistamines (first generation)	Diphenhydramine Hydroxyzine Chlorpheniramine Meclizine Doxylamine Dimenhydrinate	Block histamine	Allergy relief Induce sleep Anti-itching Antianxiety Anti–motion sickness

(Continued)

he reported that it was getting more difficult to fall asleep. Upon further questioning, the nurse practitioner discovered that Mark has been getting out of bed to pace around the room due to restless legs when he lies down. The nurse practitioner asked Mark when this started, and Mark timed the onset of symptoms to within a few weeks of having started his new digestion medication. The nurse practitioner identified that the new medication, metoclopramide, was likely triggering Mark's new RLS.

Two other classes of medications that are commonly associated with RLS are antidepressants and antihistamines. Most antidepressants can worsen RLS, particularly those that increase **serotonin** (a different neurotransmitter). Unfortunately, that means the vast majority of antidepressants can worsen RLS. Only one antidepressant, bupropion, is thought not to increase the risk of developing RLS because it does not affect serotonin levels.

The antihistamines that tend to be the biggest culprits are the older ones, such as diphenhydramine, or any of the drugs sold as "PM" medications to improve sleep. Think of it this way: if an antihistamine can make you sleepy, it can also cause RLS. Some of the new antihistamine medications will not do this. Fexofenadine, for example, does not affect the brain and should not cause RLS.

Aside from medications, people with RLS are usually counseled to avoid caffeine, alcohol, and tobacco to prevent these substances from worsening their symptoms. Alcohol is probably the most common culprit in triggering RLS among the three, but you can experiment with eliminating each of these if you don't know which ones might be your triggers. If cutting down on caffeine, alcohol, or tobacco improves your RLS, that's much better than taking extra medication to treat it. It's worth a try!

As you can see, there are plenty of reasons people might develop RLS. In addition to all of the medical conditions and medications that can trigger RLS, there is the possibility that you might have inherited a predisposition for RLS from one (or both) of your parents. The role of genetics is probably related to how your body absorbs, stores, and processes iron, but much work remains to be done to figure out all of the genetic factors in RLS. Because there are so many different conditions that can provoke RLS, it's possible for anyone to develop it now or in the future if the circumstances are right.

CHAPTER 3

What Causes RLS?

In this chapter, you will learn:

- What occurs in the brains of people with RLS
- What kinds of changes in the brain can cause RLS
- How low iron in the brain is related to all of the brain pathways in RLS

Introduction

Now that you know the types of medical conditions and medications that are commonly associated with RLS, it's time to take a deeper dive into what's going on in the bodies and brains of people with RLS. It's important to note right from the start that neuroscientists are still working out all the details, and our understanding of the causes of RLS could change based on future discoveries. What we will discuss here is the current state of knowledge of RLS.

Another caveat is that RLS might have different causes in different people. It's reasonably likely that there is no one, single explanation for all cases of RLS, so the different pathways to developing RLS might apply to some people and not others.

Fundamentals of brain structure and function

To understand the rest of this chapter, we need to start by going over the basics of how the brain works. The brain is composed mostly of two types of cells, **neurons** and **glia**. Neurons are what most people think of when they think of the brain. They're the cells that do the work that people call brain activity; they generate electrical impulses. They allow us to think, remember, see, feel, move, etc. The glia have many different functions, but you can generally think of them as the support system that keeps the neurons healthy. In the context of RLS, we're going to focus on the neurons, not the glia.

The tens of billions of neurons in the brain need a way to communicate with each other. This is where neurotransmitters come in. Neurotransmitters are chemicals that allow the neurons to send signals to each other. Some of these signals increase activity in the neuron receiving the message ("**excitatory**"), and other signals reduce activity in the neuron receiving the message ("**inhibitory**"). RLS can result if there is too much or too little activity going on in different neurons.

Dopamine, adenosine, and glutamate—Oh, my!

The neurotransmitter most closely tied to RLS is dopamine. Dopamine plays many roles in the brain and has been linked to RLS, **Parkinson's disease**, and **schizophrenia**, which all have very different symptoms.

Jeremy is a 46-year-old man who went to his primary care physician a year ago with concerns around RLS. He has been taking medication for it since then with good relief. He told his doctor that his mother had recently been diagnosed with Parkinson's disease and when she received the diagnosis from her neurologist, the doctor explained that the disease was

(Continued)

(Continued)

caused by low dopamine levels, and that she should start a medication that increased dopamine. Jeremy recognized this medication immediately as the same drug that he had been on for the past year for his RLS and is worried that he will soon develop Parkinson's disease also.

Jeremy doesn't need to worry; the fact that he takes a medication used for Parkinson's disease doesn't mean that he's destined to have it. How and why dopamine problems can cause RLS have not been completely worked out. What we do know is that the neurons that are supposed to respond to dopamine stop responding properly. Think of RLS as subscribing to satellite TV with 200 stations and having a broken satellite dish. It doesn't matter how many channels are being broadcast if you can't receive the signal. Contrast this with Parkinson's disease with lower dopamine production, as if the satellite were to stop broadcasting. There's a disruption in the signal in both conditions but for very different reasons.

People with RLS still make dopamine and sometimes even higher than normal amounts of dopamine. Most likely, RLS is caused by a problem with the dopamine **receptors** that are not processing the dopamine signal properly. Without complicating things too much, it's sufficient just to know that the end effect is that the brain's dopamine neurons are not communicating properly.

In Parkinson's disease, by contrast, the brain produces less dopamine. While there is a higher risk of RLS in people with Parkinson's disease, it's not as high as you might think. The majority of people with Parkinson's disease never develop RLS, and the majority of people with RLS do not develop Parkinson's disease.

Many of the treatments for RLS involve medications that enhance the dopamine pathway, either by supplementing dopamine directly or by stimulating the dopamine receptors. These drugs can be highly effective, but they come with risks. We'll discuss these medications more in Chapter 7.

Aside from dopamine, two other neurotransmitters have been investigated for their role in causing RLS. One of these is **adenosine**. The discovery of adenosine's role in RLS is much more recent compared to dopamine. The current understanding is that people with RLS have fewer of a certain type of adenosine receptors, which has the same effect as if the brain weren't producing adenosine. Just like with dopamine, it doesn't matter if the brain is making enough adenosine if there is no receiver on the other end to get the signal. A dysfunctional signal can sometimes be overcome if the levels of adenosine are high enough, and that's why medications that increase adenosine can be used to treat RLS.

The third neurotransmitter that has been identified as a cause of RLS is **glutamate**. Glutamate's role in the brain is to rev up many different systems throughout the brain. Unlike the low-functioning dopamine and adenosine pathways, in RLS glutamate activity is high. It is thought that high glutamate is what drives the sensation of hyperactivity that is sometimes associated with RLS (i.e., the need to move around). Drugs that reduce glutamate signals can therefore be used to treat RLS.

One more brain system involved in RLS is the **opioid** system. Many people hear opioids and think of street drugs like heroin or prescription drugs like **oxycodone**, but the brain also makes its own opioids. There is some evidence from studies on mice that problems in the opioid system can contribute to RLS.

Chan is a 36-year-old male who has been using heroin for the past 2 years. He goes to his primary care provider asking for help to stop using heroin. He tells his primary care provider that he tried to stop before, but the withdrawal symptoms were unbearable. Among the symptoms that he experienced was severe restlessness in his legs. He was unable to rest or sleep and generally felt miserable when he didn't use heroin. His primary care provider offers him buprenorphine/naloxone, a

(Continued)

(Continued)

combination medication used to help people with *opioid use disorder* to stop using heroin. Chan comes in the following week and reports that he has been able to use the new medication instead of heroin, and he has not experienced significant withdrawal symptoms.

As Chan experienced, when the brain opioid system is not working properly (in his case due to withdrawal from an external opioid), the RLS symptoms can be terrible.

The neurotransmitters involved in RLS all rely on iron in the brain to function properly. In Chapter 2, we discussed iron deficiency in depth. In brains with inadequate iron, the dopamine, adenosine, and opioid systems are less effective, while glutamate becomes too active. This is why making sure everyone with RLS has enough iron is critically important. It seems that iron deficiency may be the origin of all of these changes in the brain.

To review, there are four key systems that can function improperly in the brains of people with RLS: low dopamine transmission, low adenosine activity, high glutamate levels, and the opioid system, which interacts with the other three pathways in complex ways. These systems don't act independently. For example, one of adenosine's jobs is to reduce glutamate activity, so when adenosine goes down, glutamate goes up (Figure 3.1). Knowing about these pathways will be crucial when we discuss medications and the reasons each medication is used to help treat RLS.

Alternative theories of RLS

Although controversial, some RLS experts believe that a minority of RLS cases come from the legs themselves, instead of the brain. There's far less research on this type of RLS, but, as discussed in Chapter 2, people have been known to get RLS in just one leg after having knee

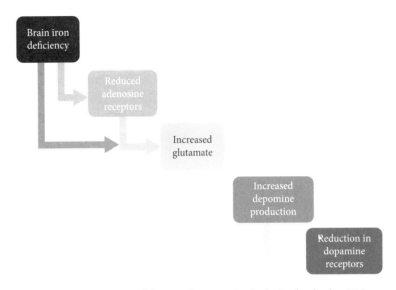

FIGURE 3.1 Diagram of changes that occur in the brain that lead to RLS.

replacement surgery, which could mean the origin of the problem is in the leg. Additionally, people with peripheral neuropathy (dysfunction in the nerves of the legs) are at higher risk of RLS. It's possible that the **peripheral nervous system** (the nerves outside the brain and spinal cord) is involved in this type of RLS. The role that iron and neurotransmitters play in the RLS symptoms in these cases is not known.

Another theory of how RLS could originate in the legs is related to low oxygen. All people have higher levels of oxygen in their chests than in their legs, but this difference is greater in people with RLS than in people without RLS. Furthermore, some of the medications we use to treat RLS, such as those that increase dopamine, also increase oxygen levels to the legs, so maybe they are so effective because they address both brain and leg causes of RLS. Similarly, regular exercise can help people with RLS, which might be because it increases oxygen in the legs. Despite these theories, most RLS providers agree that the majority (possibly the vast majority) of RLS cases originate in the brain.

Most likely, your provider will not spend much time trying to sort out different causes of your RLS other than to check your iron levels. This is because providers do not have a good way of differentiating different types of RLS, and treatment guidelines do not specify certain drugs for RLS from different causes. As a result, determining if your RLS is coming from your brain, your oxygen levels in your legs, or your nerves does not have a significant impact on your treatment options. Your RLS should be treatable even if the reason for it is never revealed.

CHAPTER 4

Consequences of RLS

In this chapter, you will learn:

- That RLS is associated with dangerous health conditions
- How RLS affects mental health
- About the impact that RLS can have on relationships

Introduction

For most conditions, one of the first questions patients ask their providers is, "Is this dangerous?" People rightfully want to know how their diagnosis will impact their health. However, for RLS, I seldom get asked this fundamental question. RLS has a reputation for being uncomfortable, but not dangerous. I think that's why patients also report that, despite mentioning their symptoms to providers for years, the sensations often receive little attention. Among all of the other health issues that primary care providers are responsible for, such as managing a plethora of chronic illnesses and arranging screening tests (e.g., **mammograms**, **colonoscopies**), restless legs just don't get very much attention.

RLS might not be as benign as we once thought, though. In the early 2000s, research started to show that RLS was associated with heart health problems. This chapter will review what's known about the link between RLS and heart disease as well as other negative health and social outcomes. The goal is not to scare you. RLS is not considered a fatal condition, but anyone with RLS ought to understand the full spectrum of its impact on the body. RLS is not just unpleasant; the evidence suggests it's also unhealthy with detrimental effects on physical, mental, and social health.

Heart disease and high blood pressure

One of the first clues that there might be an association between RLS and heart health was from research done in Sweden. From a group of 4000 men, those who reported symptoms of RLS were 1.5 times more likely to have high blood pressure and 2.5 times more likely to have other heart problems. This study was designed to assess the full spectrum of conditions that was associated with RLS, and the fact that there was a high rate of heart disease and high blood pressure was an unexpected outcome.

In a related study of 5000 Swedish women, there was an association between RLS and heart disease but not high blood pressure. These early studies simply showed an association between two conditions, and it could not be determined if the RLS caused the heart disease or high blood pressure, if said medical problems caused the RLS, or if there was some other factor causing both. This type of association is what researchers refer to as **correlation without causation**. In other words, we know they're associated, but we don't know why.

Soon after the Swedish studies, the first study of American patients looking into the association between heart disease in RLS was published. Researchers again looked at men and women who reported symptoms of RLS and found that they were more likely than those without RLS to report also having **cardiovascular disease**. Those who had more frequent symptoms of RLS also had more heart problems.

Another large study of Americans revealed an even more detailed look at this association. In this study, "heart disease" was defined broadly and included chest pain, heart attack, heart failure, and any treatment to open blocked heart arteries. Just like in the previous studies, the risk of heart disease was two to three times higher in patients experiencing RLS symptoms more nights than not. Meanwhile, people with RLS symptoms that occurred 15 or fewer times per month were not at increased risk of these heart problems. In addition, people who reported that their symptoms were more bothersome and intense were also at higher risk, indicating that the frequency of symptoms was not the only relevant factor worth examining.

Again, this is simply a correlation, and it was not yet clear from this research if RLS had a role to play in causing those heart problems. If RLS did contribute to the development of heart disease, it was not clear how, but some researchers speculated that it could be related to poor-quality sleep due to excessive movement in bed or general sleep deprivation due to difficulty falling asleep. The survey respondents with RLS did report shorter sleep times and taking longer to fall asleep at night than those without RLS, so sleep deprivation could be the missing link.

It was around this time that researchers tried to establish whether RLS was directly causing or contributing to the heart disease. For RLS to contribute to heart disease, it must develop before the heart disease. Of course, RLS predating heart disease is not proof that it causes heart disease, but at least it supports the possibility.

To investigate this issue of timing, researchers followed a group of 1986 Welsh men for 10 years. Only men who had never had a stroke or heart attack in the past were included. The men who reported having RLS were 1.67 times more likely to have a stroke during that 10-year period.

Further evidence came from a study of 70,977 women in the United States; those who had had RLS for at least 3 years were at nearly double the risk of having a nonfatal heart attack over the 6 years of the study. A separate study of 57,417 women showed that women with RLS had a 1.4 times greater risk of dying from cardiovascular disease than those without RLS, and the longer they had RLS, the greater the risk. These studies helped establish that RLS often predates heart disease and is thus a potential contributor to its development.

Not all studies have agreed with this conclusion, though. Two large studies that looked at 29,756 American female health professionals over 9 years and 19,182 American male physicians over an average of 7 years, respectively, showed no increase in cardiovascular disease, stroke, heart attack, death from cardiac causes, or need to reopen the arteries to the heart. Given that the population in these studies was all health workers, it raises the question if this is really a population that represents most people with RLS. It's possible that the RLS increased their risk of heart disease but they were able to counteract it in other ways, such as healthier diets, more exercise, or stricter adherence to prescribed medications, that would not be true of the general population. This might be why no increased risk of heart disease was seen in these studies, but it was in the others. If that theory is correct, it is all the more reason for you to eat right and exercise (more on this in Chapter 6).

The next question that had to be asked was how RLS could increase the risk for these bad health outcomes. In 2007, a study was published that looked at what happens to the blood pressures of people with RLS who also had periodic limb movements of sleep (PLMS). As we discussed in Chapter 1, many people with RLS will jerk their legs at semiregular intervals while they're sleeping, which is referred to as PLMS. This is not the same thing as RLS, but it's very common for people with RLS to do this. In the study, researchers looked to see if blood pressure went up after these leg jerks, and it did. If the leg jerks were strong enough to disturb sleep, the effect on blood pressure was even stronger.

Blood pressure is supposed to be lower when you're asleep than when you're awake. This is called the **nocturnal dip**. If your blood pressure doesn't dip at night, your body is exposed to higher blood pressure around the clock, which isn't healthy. Discovering that PLMS reduced the nocturnal dip was one of the first clues that RLS might actually have a causative impact on heart disease. This finding was replicated in 2019, and it was confirmed that people with RLS are less likely to have the nocturnal blood pressure dip.

The next hypothesis that could explain the connection between RLS and heart disease is elevated **cortisol**. Cortisol is a **hormone** released by the **adrenal gland** that increases when the body is under stress. Cortisol has a role in regulating your metabolism, your blood pressure, your blood sugar, and your sleep. If consistently high cortisol leads to higher blood pressure, elevated blood sugar, or less sleep, health problems like heart disease can develop. In the study of RLS and cortisol, cortisol was significantly elevated in patients with RLS compared to those without RLS, suggesting another mechanism by which RLS might be a contributing cause of heart disease. We also know that obesity, which can result from excess cortisol, is a risk factor for both RLS and heart disease, so this is another mechanism by which RLS might contribute to heart problems.

Third, one study showed that patients with RLS had higher leg **vascular resistance**. This means that it is harder to push blood into the legs because the arteries are tighter. Higher vascular resistance occurs for various reasons, but in the context of RLS, it could be the result of changes to the nervous system associated with the neuro- transmitter changes discussed in Chapter 3. Higher vascular resist- ance could explain why, over time, patients with RLS develop high blood pressure and heart disease.

The last question that needs to be answered to fully understand the relationship between RLS and heart disease is whether treating the RLS helps bring the risk of heart disease back down to what it is for people without RLS. One study in France looked at this question, and—good news—it does! In this study, patients who were treated for RLS showed no increased risk of either heart disease or high blood pressure. This study was relatively small and therefore not definitive, but it's certainly promising.

One reason more research has not been done to answer this ques- tion is because it requires a group of people with frequent and/or bothersome RLS to go without RLS treatment to see if they're more likely to have a bad outcome than the people who are treated. It's difficult to find enough people willing to forego treatment for years to collect this information. It would be fascinating to see if health outcomes were different depending on which medication was used for treatment, but that study has never been done.

To summarize what we know about RLS and cardiovascular disease, there is substantial evidence that people with RLS are more likely than those without RLS to have cardiovascular disease. What's less clear is why. The bulk of the research points toward RLS contributing in some way, either by raising blood pressure or by disrupting sleep. It's also possible that the changes in the body that cause RLS also cause cardiovascular disease, so RLS might not be directly to blame. If RLS does cause heart disease and high blood pressure, the good news is that you might be able to reduce your risk through healthy lifestyle choices and treating the RLS.

Depression

Depression is a serious medical condition characterized by depressed mood, loss of interest in activities that once were pleasurable, changes in appetite, and feelings of hopelessness. Also common in people with depression is a change in sleep habits, either sleeping more or sleeping less than usual. There is substantial overlap between depression and RLS. Patients with RLS are more likely to be depressed, and patients with depression are more likely to have RLS.

Some of you are probably thinking to yourselves: "I know why people with RLS are depressed; it's because living with RLS is miserable!" Certainly, the impact RLS has on someone's quality of life might play a role, but there are many things in life that can make people feel miserable. Feeling miserable doesn't mean they're going to become depressed. Depression is a medical condition; it affects people whether they can point to anything wrong in their lives or not. The changes in brain chemistry that cause depression don't care if you have a stable marriage, a well-paying job, or healthy children: depression is an illness, not a commentary on life. And just because you may be severely struggling with RLS doesn't mean you will develop depression; it takes more than struggling with the symptoms of RLS to cause depression.

Kayode is a 34-year-old male who is seeing his primary care provider for an evaluation of depression. He has felt down for much of the past 6 months. He has lost interest in things he used to find pleasurable, has been isolating himself from his friends, and generally feels hopeless. His doctor asks him about how he's been sleeping, and Kayode tells him that he has been having trouble falling asleep. He also spends much of his day in bed watching internet videos on his phone. He used to be much more active, playing tennis or going on long runs, but he hasn't done this recently. His mother finally convinced him to see his doctor. Kayode's doctor confirmed the diagnosis of depression and recommended a combination of therapy with a licensed clinical social worker and antidepressant medication.

As far back as 1965, doctors started reporting high rates of depression in patients with RLS. Subsequent research showed that people with RLS have an approximately 2.5 times higher risk of having depression than people without RLS. Just like with heart disease, this doesn't mean the RLS is the cause of the depression, but the association between the two conditions is strong. There is contradictory research on whether the severity of the RLS predicts the severity of the depressive symptoms.

After establishing the association between RLS and depression, the next step, as it was for heart disease, was to try to establish which condition develops first to explore the possibility that the RLS might be contributing to the development of depression. In a study of 56,399 women who did not have depression at the start of the study in 2002, those with RLS were more likely than those without RLS to go on to develop depression over the next 6 years. It's possible that RLS was just an earlier manifestation of another underlying condition that later also caused depression, but knowing that RLS predates depression allows for the possibility that it could contribute to causing it. At this point, we don't have research that establishes RLS as a cause of depression, only that they frequently co-occur and that having RLS puts people at higher risk for later being diagnosed with depression.

One of the logical explanations for why RLS would contribute to depression is that it reduces sleep quantity and quality, and poor sleep is known to contribute to depression. But it might be more complicated than that. In a study of patients with kidney disease (recall from Chapter 2 that kidney disease is strongly associated with RLS), those who had RLS had more depression than those with no RLS. That finding alone comes as no surprise, but they also found that the link between RLS and depression was strong even when they factored **insomnia** into the equation. That means that insomnia and the associated poor sleep quality is not the reason that the RLS group developed depression more frequently than the group without RLS; some other factor was involved.

Another study monitored the sleep of three groups of patients: those with RLS without depression, those with RLS and depression, and those with depression but not RLS. The researchers found that the two groups with RLS slept similarly to each other but different from the group with depression without RLS. Since the people with RLS slept more like each other than the two groups of people with depression, we know that the link between RLS and depression isn't just poor sleep. Once again, it appears that something other than sleep quantity or quality connects RLS and depression.

The connection between depression and RLS might have to do with the same neurotransmitter changes, such as impaired dopamine. Some of the drugs that are used to treat RLS by enhancing dopamine transmission have also been successfully used to treat depression. Although this remains speculation, it's possible that the link between depression and RLS is that they are manifestations of the same underlying problem.

> Barbara is an 83-year-old female who came to the sleep clinic seeking help for her RLS. She tells her sleep doctor that she has had mild symptoms for 40 years but never felt the need to do anything about them. Early on, she didn't even know there was a name for what she felt. Over time, she learned about RLS and quickly figured out that that's what she'd been dealing with. She goes on to tell the sleep doctor that a year ago she was diagnosed with breast cancer and underwent chemotherapy and radiation to treat it. The cancer is now in remission, she's pleased to report. However, while undergoing cancer treatment, her RLS moved from mild to severe. She says that the RLS is so bad now that it's worse than chemotherapy for her cancer. If she had to choose between more rounds of chemotherapy or getting rid of the RLS forever, she'd choose dealing with the chemotherapy over more suffering from RLS.

Barbara isn't real, but her story is. I did have a patient tell me that her RLS made her more miserable than undergoing cancer chemotherapy, and cancer chemotherapy is notoriously difficult to tolerate. I've also had multiple patients threaten to amputate their own legs if I couldn't get their symptoms under control. These patients were all absolutely miserable, but they were not depressed. I am emphasizing this point because it's important to understand that the link between RLS and depression is complicated and likely related more to brain chemistry than to the leg symptoms themselves. That means if you are concerned you might have depression (or know that you do), you should not assume that it will go away when your RLS symptoms improve. Please see your provider to address the depression directly.

A link to a free online depression screening tool is provided in the Resources and Additional Reading section at the end of the book.

Treating depression is often easier said than done, particularly in the setting of RLS. Other than the antidepressant that increases dopamine (bupropion), virtually all other antidepressants that are in common clinical practice run the risk of exacerbating RLS (see Table 2.1). This includes the **selective serotonin reuptake inhibitors (SSRIs)**, such as fluoxetine, citalopram, escitalopram, and paroxetine, which are the most common antidepressants in the United States. It also includes the **serotonin and norepinephrine reuptake inhibitors (SNRIs)**, such as the commonly prescribed drugs duloxetine and venlafaxine, and the **tetracyclic** antidepressant mirtazapine.

Older antidepressants, such as amitriptyline, are still used for various purposes, such as migraine headache prevention, but they too can exacerbate RLS. Ironically, because mirtazapine and amitriptyline are so sedating, they are sometimes prescribed as sleeping pills, but if the reason for the difficulty sleeping is RLS, this has the potential to cause more harm than good. Trazodone is another sedating antidepressant used more to treat insomnia than depression. There are reports of trazodone helping RLS and reports of it worsening RLS, so there's no clear answer for that medication.

With so many antidepressants known to make RLS worse and so many people with RLS dealing with depression, this creates a real dilemma. The depression can't be ignored, but you wouldn't want your RLS to get worse either. This situation comes up frequently. The best way to deal with this is to treat the depression independently from the RLS. While many antidepressants *can* increase RLS, that doesn't mean they *will* increase RLS, and of the two, depression is the one that is more likely to have fatal consequences. If the antidepressant worsens the RLS significantly, another one can be tried, but the depression still must take priority.

For patients with depression and RLS who have never taken an antidepressant, your provider will probably start with bupropion because it's least likely to worsen the RLS. However, not everyone does well with this medication, and if you experience side effects, be sure to discuss these symptoms with your provider. If you start any of the other medications and it exacerbates your RLS, you'll know quickly, and your provider can try something else.

The worsening of RLS can start within the first week when it's still very easy to change to another medication. At that point, it's essentially trial and error to find an antidepressant that doesn't trigger your RLS, which is almost always possible to find. And remember, no two patients will have the same results to the same medications, so be patient and discuss the benefits of your medications at every check-in.

For patients with depression and RLS who are already on an antidepressant, it is important to discuss the interaction between RLS and antidepressants with your provider. The first question to explore is how necessary you find your medication to be. Not everybody taking antidepressants needs to stay on them forever. If you think you might be able to stop your antidepressant, have a conversation with the prescriber to see if it's okay to come off it. While some people do better on long-term antidepressants, some people can safely stop them. It is always rewarding to help people get off medications they no longer need.

Patients who need to remain on an antidepressant but have never tried bupropion might be candidates to switch to bupropion to see if getting off their current antidepressant has any impact on their symptoms. However, this must be done with caution because there's a chance that the depressive symptoms get worse in the process of making this change. Another reason to make a change is if the antidepressant is no longer working well enough. Sometimes patients who have been on the same medication for years will start to feel that it isn't working as well as it did, in which case a different medication might be in order.

If your antidepressant is working well, then leave well enough alone. Your provider can manage your RLS symptoms around the antidepressant. The chances of the RLS going away by taking away an effective antidepressant are low. Since stopping your antidepressant probably won't eliminate the need for RLS medication and it could worsen your depression, it's just not worth the risk.

Anxiety

Anxiety is both a feeling and a category of mental illness. People can feel anxious without having an anxiety disorder. When the feeling of anxiety causes significant distress or impairment in functioning, that's when it becomes a disorder. Both anxiety, the emotion, and anxiety disorders are associated with RLS.

This observation was first reported in the medical journals in 1965. The authors of that report identified patients who only had worse RLS symptoms during periods of high anxiety and others who reported finding relief from RLS when going on vacation, presumably a lower-anxiety time. They concluded that anxiety was more common in patients with RLS than in the general population but recognized that RLS also occurs frequently in the absence of anxiety.

It was nearly 40 years after these early reports that the association between anxiety and RLS was formally assessed in research. One of the first studies found that there was a correlation between RLS and anxiety severity. Using a scale where scores less than 8 are considered nonanxious, 8 to 14 represents mild anxiety, 15 to 23 is moderate anxiety, and higher than 24 is severe anxiety, the subjects with RLS had an average score of 8, with about half the group scoring between 8 and 21. The subjects without RLS, by comparison, averaged 5.7 and the top half of that group scored between 5.7 and 18. This study did not collect information on the timing of the onset of symptoms, so it's not known if these patients with RLS were anxious first or had RLS symptoms first.

A large study of over 6500 subjects looked at multiple associations with RLS, and anxiety was one of the strongest. Daily RLS sufferers were 3.4 times more likely than those without RLS to have high levels of anxiety. Depression, by comparison, was only 2.2 times more likely in this study.

Looking not just at anxiety but at specific anxiety disorders, one study found that **panic disorder** and **generalized anxiety disorder** have the strongest associations with RLS. Panic disorder is a condition where people have recurrent episodes of panic attacks, which involve the sudden onset of intense feelings of fear, a sense of impending death, and physical symptoms such as sweating, chest pain, shortness of breath, and a rapid heart rate. Generalized anxiety disorder is a chronic condition involving a heightened sense of worry about everyday activities. Compared to a control group, those with RLS were nearly 5 times more likely to have panic disorder and 3.5 times more likely to have generalized anxiety disorder.

Considering cause and effect, the fact that patients report worsening of RLS when anxious implies that for at least some people, anxiety contributes to the RLS. On the other hand, the restlessness and associated difficulty sleeping and other impairments in quality of life can contribute to anxiety. There is evidence that treating RLS can reduce anxiety, lending further support to the idea that RLS increases anxiety. Likewise, certain medications, such as **benzodiazepines**, which include drugs like diazepam, lorazepam, and alprazolam, are effective for anxiety and can also be used as treatments for RLS (see Chapter 10). Overall, there seems to be a strong connection between anxiety and RLS, with the conditions interacting to exacerbate each other. It's likely that these conditions create a vicious circle.

Antidepressants are frequently used to treat anxiety disorders, not just depression, so the same information from the depression section earlier in this chapter applies here as well. For patients who use antidepressants such as SSRIs for their anxiety disorder, it is seldom sufficient treatment for the RLS to stop the medication, and it might worsen the anxiety if they do. The exception is if a new medication for anxiety is started and the response is a clear worsening of RLS. In this situation, when the connection between the drug and the symptoms is apparent, it is probably worth finding an alternative anxiety medication.

Attention deficit hyperactivity disorder

First identified in children, there appears to be an association between RLS and **attention deficit hyperactivity disorder (ADHD)** in adults as well. There is much less research on this association than on heart disease, depression, or anxiety. Two proposed explanations for this are that either RLS and ADHD share a common underlying cause or the sleep disruption caused by RLS and the associated PLMS leads to impaired daytime attention. There is also some evidence that iron deficiency might be the common link between the two as iron deficiency is a common finding in children with ADHD just like it is in patients with RLS, and iron therapy can improve both conditions. Treatment of RLS probably improves attention to some degree, but the research on this is sparse.

Dementia

Without scaring you too much, it is important to tell you that RLS has been shown to place people at increased risk for developing **dementia** (the deterioration in one or more functions of a person's brain resulting in an inability of that person to care for themselves independently). Thankfully, RLS doesn't increase your risk a huge amount. From a sample of patients over age 60 who were followed for 12 years, only 10% of them went on to develop dementia, while 6% of those without RLS developed dementia. Said another way, 90% of patients with RLS did not develop dementia over the duration of the observation time, so those are very good odds. This research was published in 2023 and was the first study to solidly establish the potential for RLS to increase the risk of dementia. For more on RLS in people with dementia, see Chapter 13.

Sleepwalking

Sleep experts do not agree on whether RLS predisposes people to sleepwalking. There is a theory that the restlessness of RLS combined with partially awakening during the night leads people to get up and walk in their sleep. There is certainly some logic to this. On the other hand, research into people who sleepwalk hasn't shown that sleepwalkers are any more likely to have RLS than anyone else. That's not to say it's impossible, but it's unlikely that if you have never been a sleepwalker, you will become one after developing RLS. More likely, there are some people who sleepwalk and a portion of them will develop RLS just by chance, but it's more of a coincidence than a cause.

Daytime sleepiness

RLS is defined by the discomfort that occurs in the evening and night, but that doesn't mean there are no symptoms the rest of the day. Nearly a quarter of all people with RLS report that they are excessively sleepy during the day. This can range from mildly unpleasant to fatal if the sleepiness leads to falling asleep behind the wheel of a motor vehicle. Daytime sleepiness can also impact job performance and lead to accidents both at work and at home. It's a serious problem and one that makes sense as a consequence of a condition that impairs people's ability to fall asleep at night.

While there are many treatments available to counteract sleepiness, the best treatment for people with daytime sleepiness related to RLS is to get the RLS under control. If the RLS is well controlled and the sleepiness persists, an evaluation for other causes of sleepiness should occur before medication to stay awake is prescribed.

The other association between daytime sleepiness and RLS is medications. It turns out that many of the medications used to treat RLS can cause daytime sleepiness as a side effect. These medications include ropinirole, pramipexole, gabapentin, pregabalin, methadone,

clonazepam, and others. We will cover these drugs in detail in
Chapters 7 to 11, but for now, it's important to know that nearly all
drugs for RLS are capable of causing sleepiness.

If these medications are taken at night when the RLS symptoms
are most active, this can be an advantage as it will help you fall asleep,
but if the drugs hang around in the body or are being used multiple
times a day, the sleepiness can become a significant problem. The
usual recommendation in this case is to switch drugs. It is not necessary to suffer from excessive daytime sleepiness as a drug side effect,
and with enough trial and error, it's likely that you and your provider
can find a treatment that is both effective and less sedating.

Relationship discord

Marriages are supposed to last through sickness and health, but RLS
can really put this vow to the test.

George is a 65-year-old male who is seeing a sleep doctor
for the first time after his primary care nurse practitioner referred him for help managing his RLS. George is accompa-
nied to the office by his wife of 15 years, Marcie. When the
sleep doctor enters the room, Marcie immediately starts the
conversation with, "Doc, you've gotta help him. He's miserable and he's making me miserable." The conversation reveals
that George keeps her awake at night by pacing around the
bedroom. When he is in bed, he moves his legs so much that
he's kicked her and worn holes in her favorite sheets. He has
stopped traveling because he can't tolerate long car rides or
flights. They can't go to a movie or the theater because he can't
sit still. She tells the doctor that she was planning to do so
many things with him, like travel, upon his retirement earlier
this year, but he won't do any of the things she wants to do
because his legs will bother him too much. On top of all that,

(Continued)

(Continued)

he's generally grumpy because he hasn't been able to sleep well, and they're fighting more than usual. He is frequently asking her to massage his legs at night when watching TV, and she's getting really tired of having to do this for him. George is frustrated because Marcie doesn't understand just how awful his legs feel; he wishes she were more sympathetic. They are both at their wits' end, all because of his RLS.

Officially, George may be the patient, but Marcie needs the doctor's help too. There's a lot of stress on this marriage because of George's condition. While sympathetic, it's hard for Marcie to understand what he's going though. She wants them to live their best lives, but at this point in time, George simply can't. Chapter 16 provides advice for caregivers in this situation.

RLS can interfere with a marriage and other close relationships in a variety of ways. If the unaffected partner doesn't understand the degree of suffering that RLS can cause, they might demonstrate a lack of sympathy, but even the most sympathetic partner is going to have limits. When the affected partner keeps the other one awake, sleep deprivation can quickly sap those emotional reserves. And it can get very frustrating when one partner wants to attend an event and the other continually nixes those plans because they require sitting.

While this didn't happen to George, another major problem that can arise in relationships is when the side effects of RLS medications begin to change behavior. For example, some of the medications used to treat RLS can induce compulsive behaviors (e.g., uncontrollable shopping, gambling, eating, or pornography consumption). It's easy to see how someone under the influence of one of these medications who gambles away the couple's life savings would create a dilemma for the partner. We will spend quite a bit more time talking about these issues in Chapter 7.

Conclusions

We don't talk much about the consequences of RLS, focusing mostly on the symptoms. RLS is such a problem in the present that it's hard to look at the future when you're just trying to get through the night. Thankfully, RLS is very treatable. Your provider can help you get this under control to minimize your risk of these complications.

CHAPTER 5

Iron Therapy

In this chapter, you will learn:

- How to increase iron in your diet
- The benefits of iron supplements for RLS
- The benefits of intravenous infusions of iron for RLS
- When to choose oral versus intravenous iron for RLS
- What to expect from iron therapy

Introduction

Brain iron deficiency is so common in RLS that everyone with symptoms of RLS should have blood tests to check for it. If your iron levels suggest that iron supplementation might help you, there are several options. This chapter will review how to increase iron in your diet, how to choose iron pills, and what to expect from an infusion of iron. There are pros and cons of these methods, and you'll learn why one might be the best choice for you.

Interpreting iron tests

In Chapter 2, you learned how complicated it can be to interpret iron levels. Recall that when your iron is checked, the tests are for ferritin and percent transferrin saturation in the *blood* even though it's the amount of iron in the *brain* that really matters for RLS. For people with RLS, if both the ferritin and percent transferrin saturation are low (ferritin < 75 µg/L and transferrin saturation < 25%), starting iron therapy is an easy decision. If just one of these two is low, though, iron therapy is still probably warranted. If both levels are above these targets or if the percent saturation is above 45%, you should think twice before supplementing iron: very high percent transferrin saturations could indicate excessive iron in the body, which could be dangerous. Further discussion with your provider and possibly additional testing would be needed to investigate that.

Dietary iron

Unless you are already taking iron pills, you are getting your iron through the food you eat. Iron in your diet comes in two forms, **heme iron** and **nonheme iron**. The difference is that heme iron comes from animals and nonheme iron comes from plants. When you eat animal flesh, the animal you are consuming has already taken nonheme iron and turned it into the form of iron your body uses (i.e., heme). When you eat iron-containing plants, your body must absorb the nonheme iron and convert it into heme iron. Nonheme iron is more difficult for your body to absorb than heme iron, so a lower percentage of the nonheme iron you eat gets into your blood. Table 5.1 provides a list of sources for both heme and nonheme iron.

While the improved absorption of heme iron sounds like a good reason for people trying to increase their iron to eat more meat, there is overwhelming evidence that higher meat intake increases the risk of many cancers. Even for people with low iron, it is healthier not to eat a diet high in red meat, and particularly processed meat (e.g., hot dogs, bacon, etc.), even though these foods would help raise iron levels. There are alternative ways—safer ways—to increase iron.

TABLE 5.1 **Dietary sources of iron**

Heme iron	Nonheme iron
Beef	Spinach
Lamb	Sweet potatoes
Pork	Broccoli
Poultry	Collard greens
Shrimp	Tofu
Clams/oysters	Fortified cereal/pasta
Liver	Dried apricots
Eggs	Beans
Sardines	Tomatoes
Tuna	Dark chocolate

Typically, a much larger quantity of nonheme iron foods must be consumed to match the iron levels of heme-iron foods.

Oral iron supplements

Some people eat a diet that is particularly low in iron, and for them, adjusting their diets to include more iron-rich foods might be enough to improve their iron levels. For many RLS patients, though, they are already eating diets that contain iron but still aren't maintaining high enough iron levels. For these people, iron supplements might be more effective. Iron pills are readily available without a prescription in pharmacies and supermarkets. In fact, there are multiple different kinds of iron pills you can buy this way, which could become overwhelming when you start shopping for them.

The most commonly recommended iron supplement is **ferrous sulfate**, but **ferrous gluconate**, **ferrous fumarate**, **ferric citrate**, and **ferric sulfate** are also available. These products might also be labeled with the word "iron" rather than "ferrous" or "ferric," so you might see "iron sulfate" or "iron citrate" on the shelf at the store; these are simply marketing differences. All of these options are nonheme iron. The most common complaint about nonheme iron supplements is constipation. They can cause an upset stomach and make your bowel movements darker. Both regular and slow-release forms are available. There is no strong argument for one or the other, so it's fair to try both and see if one causes fewer side effects than the other. You can also choose between pill and liquid forms, though liquid iron has been known to stain teeth.

Heme iron supplements are also sold, though you probably won't find them in stores outside of specialty shops. They can be purchased online but tend to be more expensive than nonheme iron pills. Heme iron is absorbed better and causes fewer digestive system side effects than nonheme iron. However, there is research indicating that high heme iron diets are linked to cancer, so there is a possibility that taking heme iron supplements could increase cancer risk. That, plus the added costs of the more expensive heme iron pills, means they are not as often recommended. No research has ever compared heme with nonheme iron supplements for the treatment of RLS, so heme iron supplements are not recommended over nonheme iron supplements.

The third type of iron you might see is called **chelated iron**. Although iron chelates are also sold as plant fertilizer, there are forms available for human consumption. Chelated iron is nonheme iron that has been modified to improve absorption and reduce side effects; at least that's what the manufacturers claim. These are designer supplements that might or might not provide the benefits they advertise, but they are probably no less effective than traditional nonheme iron pills and are thus a reasonable option. This is another area where research is lacking as no one has studied the impact of chelated versus nonchelated iron for people with RLS.

Nonheme iron is not absorbed well, but there are things that you can do to maximize absorption. First, nonheme iron should be taken with vitamin C. Vitamin C combines with iron to help your intestines absorb the iron. You can add vitamin C to your iron by buying iron pills that already contain vitamin C, taking your iron pill with a

TABLE 5.2 Foods that are recommend to eat and to avoid when taking nonheme iron supplements

Foods to eat with iron supplements	Foods to avoid with iron supplements
Oranges	Milk
Orange juice (without added calcium)	Cheese
Strawberries	Whole grains
Grapefruit	Cereals
Melon	Beans
Peppers	Nuts
	Beans
	Coffee
	Tea

vitamin C supplement, or eating or drinking high vitamin C foods and drinks when taking your iron pill.

Iron absorption can be blocked by many different foods, especially those that contain calcium. Table 5.2 lists foods that are helpful and harmful in absorbing nonheme iron. Give your iron pill a 60-minute head start before eating or drinking any of the foods on the list to avoid or else wait 2 to 3 hours after eating them to take the iron pill. Finally, it's important to keep in mind that calcium is commonly found in antacids, so if you take antacids, be sure to check the label so that you don't inadvertently mix calcium and iron pills.

Erin is a 54-year-old woman who takes no regular medications. She visits her primary care provider for a routine, annual checkup and mentions her restless legs. She tells her provider that the symptoms are bothersome but not so bad that she would want to take medication every day. Her provider suggests that they check Erin's iron levels to see if she might be a candidate for iron supplements. Erin agrees with this plan and says that if she could get the restlessness to go away with

(Continued)

(Continued)

iron, she would be happy to take the supplements. Erin's labs come back with a ferritin of 35 μg/L and a transferrin saturation of 19%, both of which are below the targets of 75 μg/L and 20%, respectively, and she starts taking iron pills.

You may hear different advice on how much iron you should take and how often to take the iron pills. There are many different expert opinions on this subject because research hasn't provided a clear, correct answer. Most of the research on iron supplements is performed on subjects with blood iron deficiency, not brain iron deficiency (the problem in RLS), and this makes a big difference because people with blood iron deficiency will absorb iron more readily than those who have low brain iron but normal blood iron concentrations. This occurs because the body uses blood iron levels, not brain iron levels, to determine how much iron it needs to pull from the intestines. That means if your blood iron is normal, you will absorb less iron because your body doesn't want to become overloaded with iron.

The best strategy for how to take oral iron in the setting of RLS is not known. Different experts recommend taking iron every other day, once a day, twice a day, or even three times per day. Once per day or once every other day is probably adequate, though. There is a risk that taking iron multiple times a day will activate the body's defense against becoming iron overloaded, which would shut down absorption of the iron. You want to take enough that the body will absorb it without taking so much that the body will start to reject it. It doesn't do you any good to take more if you're not going to absorb it anyway. Once per day is enough for many people, and more often than that will probably increase side effects.

It's important for you to understand that when you take an iron pill, only some of the pill is iron. In the case of ferrous sulfate, for example, the sulfate portion takes up some of the pill, as well as the inert material that holds the pill together. As a result, the dose listed on the front of the bottle and the amount of iron you get are not necessarily the same number. For example, a single pill of ferrous sulfate might be listed as 325 mg, but only about 65 mg of that is **elemental iron**, the pure iron that your body can utilize. Ferrous gluconate is also sold as a 325 mg pill, but that would give you only about 39 mg of elemental iron. Thus, when we discuss iron dosing, it's important to focus on the dose of elemental iron, which might only be listed in fine print on the back of the bottle. The total size of the pill is not important, only the amount of elemental iron.

A few studies have looked at oral iron supplements to treat RLS. The first one used 65 mg of elemental iron twice per day as the therapy. This dose improved symptoms, but it wasn't compared to 65 mg once a day to know if twice a day provided any benefit beyond what one pill would have done. Another study of the same twice-daily dose showed improved iron levels but no improvement in symptoms. This could be because the modest improvement in blood iron level wasn't adequate to meaningfully improve brain iron levels. The bottom line is that the optimal dose of oral iron for RLS has not yet been defined. However, 65 mg of elemental iron is a reasonable starting point. If blood iron levels do not improve on this dose, you can talk to your provider about going up to twice-daily dosing, and if there are side effects at once daily, your provider might recommend dropping the dose to once every other day.

Erin, the 54-year-old woman with mild RLS and iron deficiency who has been taking iron supplements, returns to see her primary care provider after 3 months of oral iron therapy. She tells her provider that she hasn't noticed any meaningful difference in her symptoms. Her provider confirms that she has been taking the pills properly (i.e., with vitamin C and not with calcium) and then suggests trying an iron infusion instead. Erin hesitates because she has heard bad things about iron infusions. Erin decides to hold off on an infusion for now and continue the oral iron supplements for another 3 months.

Both the provider and Erin have reasonable solutions here. Erin could try taking iron twice a day to see if that helped more than once-per-day iron or she could decide to have the infusion. Importantly, neither of them chose to give up on iron altogether. Erin still has a chance for her RLS to improve with higher levels of iron.

Intravenous iron infusions

Compared to oral supplements, much more is known about the use of intravenous (IV) iron for the treatment of RLS, and it is overwhelmingly positive. An IV iron infusion is one of the best treatments available for RLS as it improves the symptoms but also addresses the underlying cause of the RLS. No other treatment gets to the root of the problem the way IV iron does. Historically, IV iron was associated with a high rate of allergic reactions, and doctors of a certain age (like me) were trained to avoid IV iron whenever possible. Thankfully, the product causing these bad reactions (**high-molecular-weight [HMW] iron dextran**) was removed from the market in 2009 and iron infusions are now much safer.

There are several different types of IV iron: **low-molecular-weight (LMW) iron dextran, iron gluconate, iron sucrose, ferumoxytol, iron isomaltoside, and ferric carboxymaltose** (Table 5.3). Of these, most of the research on the treatment of RLS has utilized ferric carboxymaltose, but LMW iron dextran, ferumoxytol, and iron isomaltoside are all reasonable options for RLS. Conveniently, each of these four options can be safely administered in a single dose of 1000 mg, though due to packaging and insurance regulations, ferric carboxymaltose (750 mg each) and ferumoxytol (500 mg each) are often given in two doses, scheduled 1 week apart. Which of the four iron products you receive is going to be determined by which ones your provider is most familiar with and which ones will be covered by your insurance. There is no strong medical reason to go with one

TABLE 5.3 **Intravenous iron product dosing and recommendation for use in RLS**

Iron product	Dose	RLS recommendation
Ferric carboxymaltose	1500 mg once or 750 mg two doses 5–7 days apart	Recommended
Ferumoxytol	100 mg once or 500 mg two doses 5–7 days apart	Recommended
Iron gluconate	100–125 mg eight times 5–7 days apart	Not recommended
Iron isomaltoside	1000 mg once	Recommended
Iron sucrose	500 mg twice or 200 mg five times within 14 days	Not recommended
LMW iron dextran	1000 mg once	Recommended

of the four over the others, although ferric carboxymaltose is the one that most of the research has used. The other two iron products, iron sucrose and iron gluconate, on the other hand, are processed differently in the body, making them less desirable for RLS.

Generally, iron infusions are administered in an infusion center. Some of these are associated with hospitals or clinics and others are independent. Depending on the rules of the infusion center, your RLS provider might not be able to place the order for the infusion. If that's the case, you will likely be referred to a health care provider on staff or affiliated with the infusion center to have the iron infusion arranged for you. Typically, these are **hematologists** (blood doctors). Other infusion centers will allow any provider to order iron infusions directly without the need to be referred to another clinic.

Depending on the type of iron being given, the process of the infusion could be short or long. LMW iron dextran tends to take the longest to infuse because it must be administered more slowly than the others and you need a **test dose**, a small amount of medication used to check for an allergic reaction. In the amount of time between the test dose and the initiation of the rest of the infusion of LMW iron dextran, the entire dose of ferric carboxymaltose can be delivered. That being said, although each dose is quicker, only half the dose is given in 1 day, so a return trip to the infusion center is often needed for ferric carboxymaltose, while the LMW iron dextran infusion is "one and done."

When you arrive for your infusion, you might be offered **premedication** to reduce your risk of a bad reaction to the iron. While this is still a common practice that dates back to when iron infusions were more likely to cause allergic reactions, it is not necessary anymore, and it can cause more harm than good. Common premedications include antihistamines, **corticosteroids**, and **acetaminophen**. Antihistamines, themselves, can cause sedation and confusion and make RLS worse. Corticosteroids are given to reduce the risk of an allergic reaction, but the risk of an allergic reaction is so low that it is not worth the risk of a bad reaction to the corticosteroid. Acetaminophen is generally safe but serves no purpose before an iron infusion. Overall, the risks of a bad reaction to IV iron are so low that premedication is not recommended.

If you are receiving LMW iron dextran, you'll be given a test dose to see if you have an allergic reaction over the next 30 minutes before the rest of the medication is slowly infused. The actual risk of a bad reaction from LMW iron dextran is very low, but there is no harm in receiving a test dose, so it is consistently done. The other iron formulations don't require a test dose. However, ferumoxytol, like LMW iron dextran, has a **black box warning** about serious and potentially fatal allergic reactions. An allergic reaction is identified by the rapid onset of shortness of breath, wheezing, swelling, and/ or hives after receiving the medication. Should these occur, allergy countermeasures will be employed. Infusion centers have protocols to follow in these unusual scenarios. While the risk of a serious reaction is low, none these drugs should not be taken by anyone who has previously had a serious allergic reaction to IV iron. If you have had a bad reaction to iron in the past, be sure to tell your provider.

While serious allergic reactions are rare, all of the iron products can cause an **iron infusion reaction**, which is more common than an allergy. Iron infusion reactions are uncomfortable, but unlike an allergic reaction, they are not dangerous. If this occurs, you'll experience a sense of flushing, mild chest pressure, or itching. Let the nurses in the infusion center know what you're feeling so that they can stop the infusion. Symptoms tend to dissipate in a manner of minutes once the infusion is stopped, at which time the infusion can be restarted at a slower rate. If you experience an iron infusion reaction, you are still able to receive iron infusions in the future, though trying one of the other formulations (e.g., ferric carboxymaltose if you reacted to ferumoxytol) would make sense. Once the infusion is complete, assuming there were no un-expected complications, you can leave the infusion center without need for further observation or a chaperone. There are no driving restrictions after an iron infusion.

Despite flooding your blood with iron, most people don't feel resolution of their RLS right away. It will still take time for the iron to make its way into the brain. The general rule is to expect gradual im-provement over the next 4 to 8 weeks. That said, some people do feel markedly better right away, but if that doesn't happen for you, don't be discouraged because it usually takes months to get the full benefit of the additional iron. There is no need to take iron pills after receiving an iron infusion.

Some people should not get iron infusions. If you have a disorder that affects how your body stores iron, known as **hemochromatosis**, you should not get IV iron. Even without this diagnosis, if your blood iron levels show a ferritin above 300 μg/L or a transferrin saturation above 45%, you should not get IV iron. Active bacterial infections should also delay iron therapy. Certain bacteria eat iron, and the last thing you want to do would be to provide more nourishment for the bacteria you're trying to fight off. It's best to wait until after the infection clears to get the iron infusion.

If you know that you're going to need a **magnetic resonance imaging (MRI)** scan soon, you should be cautious with the timing of your iron infusion. If possible, wait until after the MRI to get the infusion; that would solve the problem. Iron is magnetic, and MRIs work using powerful magnets. An iron infusion will flood your body with so much iron that it can impair the accuracy of the MRI. How long you need to wait to get an MRI after having an infusion depends on which iron product you receive.

No firm guidelines have been established to tell you exactly how long you must wait after an iron infusion to get an MRI. Ferumoxytol is generally accepted to cause the longest delay. If possible, you should wait 3 months after the infusion for your MRI. The other iron products have a shorter timeline, with LMW iron dextran and iron isomaltoside okay at 1 month and ferric carboxymaltose at 1 week. If the MRI is too urgent to wait out this length of time after having an infusion, it's best to just get the MRI, but you should mention the recent infusion to the provider ordering the MRI to help make that decision. These timelines are provided for the ideal scenario when you have the time to wait.

Choosing between oral and IV iron

IV iron is overall better for the treatment of RLS than oral iron. That doesn't mean that everyone with RLS should start with IV iron. IV iron is much more costly and comes with more risks than oral iron. Also, some people just hate needles. Therefore, oral iron is the better initial option for some people.

The most important factor in determining oral versus IV iron for initial therapy is the ferritin level. Intuitively, you might think that if the level of iron is really low, an infusion would be better, but it's actually the opposite. The lower your ferritin, the better your body will absorb oral iron. Once ferritin levels get above 50 µg/L, your body will start reducing how much oral iron it absorbs. When people with normal blood iron need to get extra iron to correct their brain iron deficiency, IV iron is going to be more effective. For people with both blood and brain iron deficiency, though, oral iron might work just fine.

A convenient way to remember when to choose IV over oral iron is the four I's:

Intolerant	If you have side effects from oral iron, consider IV iron.
Intensity	If you have severe RLS and don't want to wait for oral iron to bring your iron levels up, consider IV iron.
Ineffective	If you have tried oral iron and have not seen improvements in your iron levels or your symptoms, consider IV iron.
Inflammation	If you have a ferritin level between 100 and 300 µg/L and a transferrin saturation below 20%, consider IV iron.

Some people have a difficult time tolerating the side effects from oral iron, and for them, IV iron is usually much easier to tolerate. You can also consider speed when choosing oral versus IV iron. IV iron is simply a faster way to get your iron levels up, which is important for people with intense symptoms. Another reason to go for the infusion instead of the pills is if you have already tried iron pills and they haven't worked or wouldn't be expected to work.

The fact that iron pills did not improve your RLS does not mean that an Iron infusion won't help. For people who have had certain procedures, such as weight loss surgery, you have lower odds of absorbing oral iron well, and IV is likely the better option. Finally, inflammation causes ferritin levels to go up, which causes absorption of iron to go down. Thus, if your body is inflamed and you have a high ferritin with a low transferrin saturation, you're likely to benefit more from IV than from oral iron.

Erin is back for another 3-month checkup. Her legs are no better after taking oral iron twice per day for the past 3 months. She has done some reading online and spoken to her friend who had an IV iron infusion and decided that she would like to proceed with an infusion herself. Her primary care provider orders updated iron labs. Erin's ferritin is now 65 µg/L with a transferrin saturation of 21%. Her provider agrees that an IV iron infusion is warranted, and a one-time infusion of LMW iron dextran, 25 mg as a test dose followed by a one-time infusion of 975 mg with no premedication, is ordered. Erin ends up doing very well with her infusion with no side effects. Within about a month, her RLS symptoms improve enough that she no longer thinks about them on a nightly basis.

Follow-up testing and additional iron

After beginning oral iron therapy, iron testing should be repeated in about 12 weeks. At that point, dosing adjustments can be made if needed. If there has been no improvement in blood iron levels, proceeding to an IV iron infusion is a reasonable next step. For those who have received an iron infusion, you should have your iron levels rechecked after about 8 weeks. This test should take place even if you are feeling better because it's important to know what blood level of iron corresponds to improvement in your symptoms. And if you aren't feeling better, it is important to ensure that the infusion got your blood levels to a high enough level. After 8 more weeks, iron levels can be checked again to ensure that they are stable. If iron levels drop between the first and second 8-week periods, additional testing might be needed to figure out why your body is losing iron so quickly.

This could potentially include a **colonoscopy** to see if you are losing blood from your intestines.

There is no specific timeframe after one iron infusion to repeat the infusion. Some people never get a second one. But if the first infusion works and then symptoms return in the future, iron levels should be rechecked. If your iron has dropped, an infusion can be repeated. You are eligible for a repeat infusion with a ferritin less than 300 μg/L and a transferrin saturation less than 45%, assuming your iron numbers have dropped since the initial 8-week mark after the first infusion. If your symptoms worsen and your iron levels have not dropped from the initial postinfusion labs, other causes of the exacerbation should be considered before receiving more iron.

Iron in perspective

Iron supplementation, especially IV iron infusions, is highly effective in the treatment of RLS, but it doesn't work immediately, it doesn't last forever, and it doesn't work for everyone. While anyone with low iron and RLS should be treated to get their iron levels up, this is only one strategy to improve RLS symptoms. The next several chapters will address both nonprescription and prescription therapies that can be used in conjunction with iron therapy. It's very likely that one or more of these strategies will work for you!

CHAPTER 6

Treatment of RLS Without Prescription Drugs

In this chapter, you will learn:

- Techniques to stimulate your legs to reduce your RLS
- Strategies for diet and dietary supplements to improve RLS
- Light and electrical devices for RLS
- The importance of exercise for RLS

Introduction

Any time you can safely avoid taking more medications, you probably should. If your RLS is mild, you might be looking for a way to treat your symptoms that avoids prescription drugs. Or maybe you're already taking a medication, and you don't want to increase the dose but your legs are still somewhat restless. In either case, you might benefit from the drug-free strategies in this chapter. Generally speaking, the options can be broken down into techniques to stimulate your legs, dietary changes and over-the-counter supplements, devices and wraps, and exercise.

This chapter will review different strategies that are frequently employed as home remedies along with some prescription therapies that don't involve medication. The US regulatory system allows for supplements, devices, and procedures to be on the market with less evidence that they are effective than would be acceptable for medications. Thus, many of the topics in this chapter will have little high-quality research supporting their use. Even so, many medication-free treatments for RLS have been used for long enough that providers have a good sense of which ones are most effective.

Counterstimulation

Counterstimulation is a general category of RLS treatments that share the concept of providing sensory stimulation to the legs. In short, they give your brain something else to process instead of the restless sensations.

Temperature

Heat, such as from hot baths or using a hot tub, is one form of counterstimulation. People who use hot water to ease their RLS symptoms often describe needing the water to be nearly scalding hot to be effective, so if you choose this method, you must be careful not to burn yourself. Further, spending excessive time in a hot tub can cause health risks, such as excessively low blood pressure or lung problems from inhaling the vapors from the chemicals used in sterilizing the hot tub. Because of these risks, this option is only viable for short durations.

Another problem with hot water therapy is that it's not a strategy that can be employed while in bed. It can calm your legs while you're in the bath, but unless you fall asleep quickly after drying off, your restlessness might return before you are down for the night. Heating pads, which also offer heat therapy, don't seem to work as well, while also placing you at risk for severe burns if you fall asleep with one on.

While less common than heat therapy, some patients have used ice baths (one patient of mine refers to it as his "slushie"). If this works for you, that's great, but again, be careful not to get so cold that you

hurt yourself in the process. Overall, heat (or ice) is a viable way of reducing RLS symptoms. Unfortunately, it is not always sufficient, and
many people who use thermal therapies also use other prescription or
nonprescription strategies.

Grace is a 51-year-old woman who has had severe RLS for
many years, and for the past 5 years, she has been under the
care of a sleep physician to treat her symptoms. As part of her
treatment, she received an intravenous (IV) iron infusion with
good results. She also took nightly prescription medication
to control her symptoms. At her most recent visit with her
sleep physician, she reported that she had intestinal bleeding,
causing her iron levels to drop, and she ran out of her medication, leading to a return of horrible restlessness in her arms
and legs. Awaiting her appointment in the sleep clinic, she has
been managing the best she could by taking very hot baths
at night, which is the only thing she has found to reduce her
symptoms.

Touch

Tactile stimulation, including massage, vibration, and compression, is a form of counterstimulation that is both safe and effective.
You can use massagers or a compassionate partner to help you rub
your legs. Sometimes just flipping over in bed will change the pressure on your legs and improve your RLS. For other people, the opposite is true and lying on their back is better. Weighted blankets
have helped some patients keep pressure on their legs during the
night. A vibrating pad was sold as a means of generating stimulation to the legs while in bed, but it is currently off the market due
to poor sales.

Squeezing the legs tends to help many people with RLS. **Sequential
compression devices** (also known as **pneumatic compression devices**

as they use air to create compression), most frequently used in the medical setting to help prevent blood clots in hospitalized patients, have been studied for RLS with good results. The price of these for home use can vary quite a bit, with some selling for up to $800, but more affordable options are available. These can be purchased without a prescription.

A less costly option would be **compression stockings**, which are readily available in most pharmacies, but they don't tend to squeeze as much as pneumatic compression and may not be as effective. Additionally, not everyone can tolerate them. The itching, sweating, and pain they can cause may limit their use for some people.

There is one prescription-only counterstimulation device that is marketed for the treatment of RLS: **Restiffic**. Restiffic is a foot wrap that provides stimulation to pressure points in the feet to help relieve restlessness. They come in three sizes based on shoe size. You can't walk while wearing them, and the manufacturer warns against using them if you have poor circulation, varicose veins, neuropathy, blood clots in your legs, swelling in your legs, any breaks in your skin or bruising, diabetes, heart failure, kidney failure, or pregnancy. Given that many of these conditions are commonly associated with RLS, Restiffic is not an option for a large number of people who suffer from RLS. However, for the right person, Restiffic might reduce the need for prescription medication. At the time of this writing, a pair of Restiffic foot wraps costs $99 and is only available in the United States.

Distraction

Sometimes just getting your mind off your legs is enough to reduce your symptoms. Knitting, doing puzzles, or otherwise engaging the mind more than you typically would with activities like watching TV can be beneficial for some people. And at least one of my patients has reported that sexual arousal and sexual activity reduced his RLS at night. Since many people associate sexual activity (with or without a partner) with better-quality sleep at night, there are likely several benefits to this approach.

Diet and supplements

Many patients report that certain foods exacerbate their RLS. In Malcolm's case, it was carbohydrates. Different people are sensitive to different foods, so treating your RLS with a specific diet will require some trial and error. Commonly reported food triggers include carbohydrates (especially those that are high in sugar), fried foods, and salty foods. There are lots of tasty foods in those groups, for sure, but if avoiding some of them can relieve your RLS, it's probably worth it to make the dietary sacrifice. Caffeine-containing drinks are well known to worsen RLS; chocolate also contains caffeine, making chocolate (caffeine + sugar) a common trigger. Surprisingly, some people do fine with sugar and find that artificial sweeteners are their trigger instead. You should be able to experiment with this to figure out if real or fake sugar is worse for your legs.

Malcolm is a 72-year-old man having a routine health maintenance visit with his primary care nurse practitioner. As part of his visit, the nurse practitioner advised him to lose weight, and he recommended that Malcolm try a low-carbohydrate diet. Malcolm also reported during the appointment that he was having restless feelings in his legs at night that were keeping him awake. The nurse practitioner prescribed him medication to take until he was able to see a sleep physician and provided him a referral to a sleep medicine clinic. Two months later, he arrived at the sleep clinic and told the sleep physician that he never filled the prescription for RLS medication. He was pleased to report that avoiding carbohydrates has reduced his restlessness at night and he was doing well enough that he debated whether or not he even needed the appointment at all anymore.

While food triggers that worsen RLS have been relatively well described, less is known about foods that can help reduce RLS symptoms. The general principle when it comes to a healthy RLS diet is that you want foods that reduce inflammation. This can include tart cherries (and tart cherry juice), leafy green vegetables, berries, nuts, and beans. Colorful, natural, and unsweetened foods are your best bets.

Supplements

Magnesium

Magnesium is a dietary supplement that is commonly tried by patients with RLS. Several research studies have attempted to determine if magnesium is effective in treating RLS, and the results have been mixed. While reasonably safe, experience shows that magnesium is not likely to help much, if at all. If it did, there would be far fewer people still suffering from RLS out there. It is not recommended to check magnesium levels in everyone with RLS, but if you are found to be deficient of magnesium for other reasons and you also have RLS, it is possible that supplementing magnesium will relieve some of the restlessness. Most people are not deficient in magnesium, though, and supplementing magnesium is not expected to help you if you aren't deficient.

Vitamin D

Vitamin D supplementation has been shown to benefit some people with RLS. All of the major neurotransmitters involved in RLS (dopamine, glutamate, and adenosine—see Chapter 3) are associated with vitamin D. Research has linked low vitamin D levels to having RLS and taking vitamin D supplements to improvement in RLS. Whether vitamin D supplements help people with RLS who are not deficient in vitamin D is unknown, though. For people who do have low vitamin D levels, supplementation is recommended regardless of whether or not they have RLS, and the good news is that those who do have RLS might see improvement in their symptoms as an added benefit.

Although it is not yet considered standard for everyone with RLS to have their vitamin D level checked, this will probably become more common as more is discovered about this association. Other vitamins, including vitamins B_6, B_{12}, C, E, and folic acid, have all been reported as effective in very small groups of people with RLS, but there is so little research on these that no recommendations can be made.

Proprietary supplements

A variety of **proprietary blends** of herbs and supplements are marketed for the treatment of RLS. It is impossible to review them all due to the sheer number of them, but there are some general guidelines to follow when considering taking them. With regard to safety, keep in mind that "natural" is not the same as "safe." Mercury, cyanide, and arsenic are all natural, but you ingest them at your peril. A product that advertises itself as a natural alternative to medication isn't necessarily safer than prescription medications. Quality controls are much stronger for prescription pills than for less regulated supplements. What is listed on the bottle of a supplement might not be what is inside the bottle.

Some proprietary supplements contain a combination of vitamins and minerals. These are probably safe, and you can follow the guidance provided in this chapter for each individual vitamin and mineral when choosing one of those. For the ones that contain herbs, it is important to discuss these with your physician. Certain herbs can damage your liver or kidneys, or they can interact with other medications you might be taking. Keep in mind that if an herb has an effect on your body, it's functioning as a drug, and your medical team should be aware of these and all other over-the-counter supplements that you are taking.

Cannabidiol

In the last few years, there's been a substantial increase in the availability of **cannabidiol (CBD)** products. Providers are now asked about CBD for treating a wide variety of conditions, including RLS, on a regular basis. The only study to investigate CBD for RLS showed no significant improvement in symptoms. Thus, it is not recommended. There are published reports of **cannabis (marijuana)** being used by patients to treat their RLS effectively but no formal research. The primary difference between CBD and cannabis is that cannabis contains hundreds of chemicals, including **tetrahydrocannabinol (THC)**; CBD is just one of these chemicals. THC can also cause intoxication and hallucinations, and without further research into the full risks and benefits of regular use for RLS, it is not recommended.

Devices

Near-infrared light therapy

A unique approach to treating RLS is the use of **near-infrared light therapy**. Infrared light is invisible to humans; near-infrared light is the portion of infrared light that is just outside of our visual range. Manufacturers of near-infrared light devices make many claims about what they can treat (joint pain, muscle injury, bone disorders, strokes, traumatic brain injuries, skin disorders, eczema, wrinkles, and baldness, to name a few). Anything that claims to treat so many conditions should be approached with healthy skepticism.

Research on near-infrared light therapy for RLS dates back to 2010, but the studies have been small and don't always utilize a **placebo** (an inert, sugar pill), so skepticism is still warranted. The proposed mechanism by which near-infrared light could improve RLS is by stimulating growth of new blood vessels in the legs. Theoretically, the more blood flow (and more oxygen) there is in the legs, the better the legs should feel. An alternative explanation is that the light stimulates production of chemicals in the legs that increase blood flow through existing blood vessels, with the end result also being more oxygen in the legs. These theories are plausible; they're just not studied enough to know if they're correct.

Although generally considered safe, near-infrared therapy is not without risks, and the risks increase with increased exposure. Excessive infrared light exposure could cause skin irritation or damage or eye redness or even, in extreme cases, cataracts. The jury is still out on this potential therapy, which is neither readily available for most people nor covered by insurance.

Susan is a 73-year-old woman with a longstanding history of RLS. She has been seen in the general neurology clinic for many years and has tried several different medications for her RLS but had side effects from all of them. At today's visit at the neurologist's office, she hands the physician assistant she is seeing an article she printed from a website describing a way of treating RLS without medications. She asks the physician assistant if she can try it instead of trying another pill. Susan's internet sleuthing turned up near-infrared light therapy as a treatment option for RLS. She'd never heard of it before, but she was intrigued by the fact that it offered a drug-free cure. Her natural skepticism led her to wonder if it was too good to be true, but she figured she would ask her neurologist just in case it was an option for her. The physician assistant answered honestly that he has never heard of this treatment before and wouldn't know how to obtain it for her.

Tonic Motor Activation system

A recent development is the US Food and Drug Administration–cleared device called a **tonic motor activation (TOMAC) system**. This device is still under development and not yet on the market at the time of this writing. It has shown promise in early trials, though. This treatment is designed for people with moderate to severe RLS for whom medications have not fully controlled symptoms. The device consists of a pair of straps that wrap around the lower leg and use electrical stimulation to activate the **peroneal nerve**. Stimulation of this nerve causes a sustained contraction in the calf muscles with the goal of allowing you to sleep better while wearing them. This product will likely be on the market by the time you read this, but it is not yet sold at this time, and pricing information is not available.

Transcutaneous electrical nerve stimulation units

In the meantime, electrical stimulation using a device called a **transcutaneous electrical nerve stimulation (TENS) unit** has not been formally studied for use in RLS, but there are anecdotes suggesting that it might be effective. If TENS units are effective, it's not clear if this is due to counterstimulation (i.e., the sensation of electricity distracts from the restlessness) or if the electrical stimulation is changing the nervous system or blood circulation in a way that fundamentally counteracts the RLS. These devices are available over the counter and have a favorable safety profile.

Repetitive transcranial magnetic stimulation

Using magnets to treat brain diseases began in the 1980s, and today it is most commonly associated with the treatment of clinical depression. **Repetitive transcranial magnetic stimulation (rTMS)** is a procedure that uses magnetic pulses directed at specific areas of the brain to disrupt activity in that region of the brain. Based on the idea that parts of the brain are overactive in people with RLS, researchers tried rTMS as a possible treatment. In one study, in which the participants had 14 sessions of rTMS over a period of 18 days, RLS severity was cut in half. Other studies have shown similar benefits. Unfortunately, this treatment is not currently available outside of a research setting. rTMS is not approved for RLS therapy, and it would be difficult, if not impossible, to find someone who will perform this procedure for you, likely at a very high out-of-pocket cost.

Acupuncture

Acupuncture is a traditional Chinese medicine practice that dates back thousands of years. Like near-infrared light therapy, it has been used to treat a plethora of conditions. Unlike near-infrared light therapy, though, there is substantial research supporting its benefits in many conditions, such as pain management and headache reduction. The research on acupuncture for RLS is not particularly robust, but there are two studies that have shown it to be beneficial. One study showed that it was useful as a supplement to prescription medication, while another showed that it was useful as an independent therapy. The risks of acupuncture are low when administered by reputable and well-trained acupuncturists, but there is not enough research on this treatment to make a recommendation about its use for people with RLS.

Sclerotherapy

For people with **varicose veins, sclerotherapy** might be an option to reduce RLS symptoms. Varicose veins are large and twisted veins, typically in the legs, that can cause pain with prolonged standing due to the effect of gravity on blood circulation. Not much is known about how frequently RLS occurs in people with varicose veins, which are very common. A small study from 1995 found that treating the varicose veins using sclerotherapy reduced RLS symptoms, with recurrence of RLS in only 28% of the people who received the treatment after a period of 2 years.

Sclerotherapy is a relatively minor procedure in which a chemical solution is injected into the varicose vein, causing it to close and route blood through healthier veins instead. It can be difficult to know if your RLS is related to your varicose veins or completely independent. Sclerotherapy will only help you if your RLS is coming from the veins.

If you have varicose veins, your RLS only occurs after long days on your feet, and your legs ache significantly at the end of the day, you might find sclerotherapy beneficial. This procedure is typically performed in **vascular surgery** clinics, and your primary care or sleep medicine provider can make a referral for you.

Exercise

Many people with RLS say their legs feel worse at night when they've exercised too much. Many others say that their legs feel worse at night if they've been too sedentary all day. So which is it? It's both. If you're generally a sedentary person, getting more active with a moderate-intensity, aerobic exercise program is likely to help your RLS. It's also likely to help your sleep in general, not to mention your overall mental and physical health. On the other hand, intense exercise, especially later in the day, can trigger RLS. Consistency seems to be important also. Getting a lot more or a lot less exercise in a given day can worsen RLS that night.

If aerobic exercise is not for you, there is research supporting stretching exercises, and lower body strength or resistance training can also be beneficial. For example, one study looked at a combination of walking on a treadmill for 30 minutes at a pace brisk enough to increase the participants' heart rates and resistance training designed for people who had never lifted weights before. After completing these exercises 3 days per week for 6 weeks, there was a 39% reduction in RLS severity. This is a relatively small time commitment for a pretty big gain.

After implementing some of these nonprescription strategies, you might still require medications to control your symptoms, but you might be able to take a lower dose, which can greatly reduce your risk of side effects. Some of these strategies may become the mainstays of therapy as we learn more about them. There is much hope for the future!

CHAPTER 7

Dopamine Agonists for RLS

In this chapter, you will learn:

- Which medications are considered dopamine agonists and how they are used
- What are common side effects of dopamine agonists and their withdrawal symptoms
- What are tolerance and augmentation
- What are impulse control disorders
- How to discontinue dopamine agonists

Introduction

In Chapter 3, we reviewed the neurotransmitters that are involved in causing RLS, including dopamine, adenosine, and glutamate. The next few chapters will take that information a step further and discuss how medications can affect these neurotransmitters and relieve RLS. In many cases, RLS providers knew these medications helped reduce restlessness but didn't understand why or how until more research uncovered the roles of these neurotransmitters. Knowing which drugs could effectively treat RLS was helpful in discovering the causes of RLS. Furthermore, understanding the underlying changes in the brain that cause RLS led doctors to explore potential treatment options from among existing drugs that impact those brain systems.

TABLE 7.1 **Dopamine-related medications for RLS**

Generic name	Brand name	Class	Route	Generic available
Carbidopa/levodopa	Sinemet	Dopamine replacement	Oral	Yes
Ropinirole	Requip	Dopamine agonist	Oral	Yes
Pramipexole	Mirapex	Dopamine agonist	Oral	Yes
Rotigotine	Neupro	Dopamine agonist	Skin patch	No

Working back and forth, brain scientists and brain doctors have discovered multiple options to treat RLS. Over the next several chapters, we will review the pros and cons of these options and discuss how providers end up choosing one of these over another. Medications will be referred to using their generic names, but you might know them by their brand names, which are included in Table 7.1.

This chapter will start the discussion of prescription drug therapy for RLS with medications that affect dopamine. We will cover the history of these drugs and how they are used in clinical practice. Very important information about the side effects and risks of these drugs will be included, along with strategies you and your health care provider can use to help you stop these medications if necessary.

History

We will start our discussion of medications with **ropinirole**, the first drug to be approved by the US Food and Drug Administration (FDA) for RLS. Ropinirole is a dopamine **agonist**, which means that it attaches to and activates neurons with dopamine receptors on them. Ropinirole was first approved for the treatment of Parkinson's disease in 1997. Given what was known about the role of dopamine in RLS, researchers repurposed ropinirole for RLS and reported positive findings in 2001. Additional studies led the FDA to approve ropinirole for RLS in 2005. Ropinirole rapidly became the standard of care for RLS, and it is still what many physicians think of first when they think of RLS.

Prior to the development of ropinirole, the common therapy for RLS was **carbidopa and levodopa**, two medications that are used together, primarily to treat Parkinson's disease. Unlike ropinirole, which attaches to dopamine receptors but does not actually create dopamine, levodopa is directly converted to dopamine in the brain and thus functions as a dopamine replacement for people whose brains do not otherwise make enough of it. Carbidopa/levodopa is still used for RLS, though far less frequently than it was just 20 years ago.

Ropinirole was not the first dopamine agonist on the market, but it is less toxic than those that came before it. Those drugs, **bromocriptine** and **pergolide**, have different chemical structures than the more modern dopamine agonists, and they are not in regular circulation in the US for RLS anymore. Ropinirole is also not the last dopamine agonist to hit the market. The year after ropinirole was approved, a closely related drug, **pramipexole**, was labeled for use in RLS. Ropinirole is still somewhat more commonly prescribed, but both are mainstays in RLS therapy. A third drug, also very closely related to ropinirole and pramipexole, called **rotigotine**, received its FDA approval for RLS in 2008. While ropinirole and pramipexole are taken as pills, rotigotine is delivered through a patch placed on the skin.

The three dopamine agonists in use today, ropinirole, pramipexole, and rotigotine, share a very important quality: they work! It is very likely that your RLS will improve if you start one of these medications. Other advantages include the simplicity of taking the medicine in pill form (for ropinirole and pramipexole) and the cost (typically less than $10/month for the pills). Rotigotine patches, which are not yet available as a **generic**, might be preferable to pills for some people, but they do not share the benefit of cost, are not often covered by insurance plans, and can run hundreds of dollars per month even with insurance coverage in some cases.

Another benefit of dopamine agonists is that these are not particularly toxic drugs. No monitoring of your liver, kidney, heart, or lung function is needed while taking them, which means no regular blood draws are required. From that perspective, they have a very favorable safety profile.

Nils is a 41-year-old man with multiple sclerosis who is seeing his neurologist for a routine visit. He mentions that he is still bothered by RLS even after stopping caffeine and alcohol consumption. He recently had his iron levels checked at his primary care provider's office, and they were sufficient. Nils told his neurologist that he would like to try a prescription medication to get some relief from his RLS. His neurologist prescribed pramipexole 0.125 mg nightly and asked Nils to let him know if he had any side effects.

Dosage

When starting a dopamine agonist, it's important to start with a low dose to minimize the risk of side effects. The goal is to find the lowest possible dose that still works to control your symptoms. For ropinirole, that usually means starting at 0.25 mg and for pramipexole that means 0.125 mg. Your provider will likely begin by prescribing one pill per night to be taken before your symptoms typically start. If you suffer from RLS all evening, don't wait until bedtime to take your medicine. If you find that the medication wears off too quickly, extended-release versions of the pills are available. If you only have occasional RLS symptoms, it is okay to use these medications on an as-needed basis. For example, you might only take a pill before getting on an airplane or watching a movie. That's fine if that's all you need.

TABLE 7.2 **Common doses of dopamine agonists for RLS**

Generic name	Starting dose	Dose adjustments	Maximum recommended dose
Ropinirole	0.25 mg per night for 2 nights then 0.5 mg	0.5 mg per week	4 mg per night
Pramipexole	0.125 mg per night	0.125 mg per 4-7 days	0.5 mg per night
Rotigotine	1 mg per 24 hours	1 mg per week	3 mg per 24 hours

Although your provider will tailor your medication dose to suit your symptoms, there are recommended maximum dosages of 4 mg of ropinirole, 0.5 mg of pramipexole, or 3 mg of rotigotine when these drugs are used for RLS. Table 7.2 provides common dosing strategies for RLS. Although higher doses are recommended for Parkinson's disease, the brains of people with that condition make less dopamine than people with RLS and thus require different doses of medication. If you have moderate kidney disease or are on kidney dialysis, your maximum dose might be lower, especially if you're taking pramipexole. If you have liver disease, you can usually take these medications without adjusting the doses.

Nils follows up with his neurologist 3 months later, stating that he had no side effects from the pramipexole but that it only provided about 30% relief from his RLS. He asked his neurologist for something more effective. His neurologist recommended increasing the dose to 0.25 mg and told Nils if that wasn't enough, he could increase to 0.5 mg. Three months later, Nils returns and reports that his RLS is doing very well on 0.5 mg. He continues to report no side effects.

Side effects

As effective as dopamine agonists are, they are far from risk free. There are both short-term and long-term concerns with these medications. The list of potential risks is the same for all three medications, with the caveat that the rotigotine patch can also cause skin irritation, which the pills won't do. The list of potential risks is also quite long, and we will not cover every possible risk or side effect in this chapter. Comprehensive lists of known risks and side effects are available from your provider or online. The resource list at the end of this book can help guide you to reliable online references for this information.

The most common side effect of dopamine agonists is nausea. This doesn't always last, and many people will get over the initial nausea and then tolerate the medication well. Another relatively common side effect is lightheadedness, particularly if you stand up quickly. These drugs can also cause sleepiness. If that only occurs at night, it might not bother you, but if it starts to affect you in the daytime, it's a problem. Not only can you feel generally drowsy, but also the medications are known to cause sudden, unexpected episodes of falling asleep. This can be dangerous, especially if it happens while you're driving.

A frightening side effect experienced by a minority of people taking dopamine agonists is **hallucinations** (seeing, hearing, or feeling things that aren't really there). This tends to be more of a problem at the dosage levels used in Parkinson's disease than the lower doses used for RLS, but some patients with RLS wind up on very high doses and can experience this.

Of the oral dopamine agonists, pramipexole is more likely to cause hallucinations, but ropinirole is more likely to cause lightheadedness and sleepiness. There isn't much research comparing ropinirole to pramipexole head to head, but one study found that patients taking pramipexole had better symptom control and fewer side effects than those on ropinirole, suggesting that between these relatively similar drugs, pramipexole probably has the edge but not by much. There is no research directly comparing rotigotine to the others.

> Nils has now been on pramipexole 0.5 mg for a year. At his next follow-up visit with his neurologist, he reports that for the past month, it has not felt as effective as it was when he first started it. Remembering how much better he felt when he went from 0.25 mg to 0.5 mg, he requests another dose increase from his neurologist. She prescribes 1 mg pills. Nils tries the stronger pills that night and once again has a great night of sleep.

Complications

Most people who start a dopamine agonist for RLS feel better very quickly, and most experience none of the possible side effects. Sounds great, right? Unfortunately, even if you tolerate the medication well, there are long-term effects to consider. One problem with the dopamine agonists is that many people will develop **tolerance** to them. That means that the effective dose you started on becomes less effective over time. Nils from the vignette is experiencing tolerance. If you mention to your provider that the medication isn't helping as much as it used to, your dose might get increased. If that happens, you'll likely feel better again very quickly. This can develop into a continuous cycle, though. The longer you are on the medication, the more you need to take to get the same effect. This is how people go from being on the lower RLS-range doses to the higher Parkinson's disease–range doses.

Higher doses mean higher risk of side effects. Maybe you didn't have sleepiness or hallucinations at the lower doses, but you might develop them as your dose goes up. Then what? Now you're on a high dose of medication, it's not working all that well anymore, and you have side effects. This is—I hate to say—extremely common.

Six months later, Nils returns, and his neurologist immediately notices a change. He looks tired and stressed out. Nils explains that he has not been getting much sleep lately because he has been staying up late playing online poker. He lost his job after not showing up for work three times in the past 2 months. He feels like his life is falling apart. When asked about his RLS, he tells his neurologist that when he takes the medication at night, he's fine, but by morning, when he's sitting at his computer playing poker, his legs start acting up again. He asks if he can add in a morning dose of pramipexole to handle the morning symptoms.

Even at moderate doses, dopamine agonists place you at long-term risk of developing an **impulse control disorder (ICD)**. ICDs are scary. Essentially, an ICD means that if you have an impulse to do something, you do it. There is no brake that tells you to stop doing what you're doing even if it's harming you. There are four classic ICDs associated with dopamine agonists: shopping, gambling, eating, and sex/pornography. All of these can be considered acceptable behaviors in moderation, but people with an ICD do these to extremes. They might gamble for 24 hours straight despite losing money they cannot afford to lose (like Nils). They might start shopping online, buying gifts for everyone they know, going into debt to do so. They might start compulsively consuming pornography, not stopping to take care of personal hygiene or social obligations. All of these things happen, and they are devastating to the people who endure them.

The best defense against ICDs is to keep the dose of medication as low as possible. It seems to take at least 0.5 mg of pramipexole, for example, before an ICD can set in. With ropinirole and rotigotine it's less clear that dose matters as much, but there is still probably some higher risk with higher doses. The second-best defense is knowledge.

Knowing about ICDs doesn't prevent them, but they help you and your family members recognize what is going on quickly so the drug can be stopped before years of harm have occurred. Everyone taking a dopamine agonist needs to be aware of this potential complication and report it to the prescribing provider if it develops. Fortunately, ICDs aren't common at the usual RLS dose range, so most people on appropriate doses will never go through this.

The more common long-term problem with dopamine agonists is **augmentation**. Up to 30% of patients who take dopamine agonists will develop augmentation, which is a worsening of symptoms due to the drugs themselves. Augmentation can set in within months of starting a dopamine agonist or after years of taking them. You'll recognize augmentation if it happens to you because you'll start to have your RLS symptoms earlier in the day or in parts of your body, like your arms, that weren't previously affected.

RLS is a condition that worsens at night; it's not common for people to have severe symptoms during the day. Severe daytime symptoms are a common manifestation of augmentation from dopamine agonists. Augmentation can also manifest as having symptoms sooner after sitting down or as your medications taking longer to provide relief. Nils from the vignette has augmentation (he is having morning symptoms) in addition to a gambling ICD.

Some aspects of your RLS care might make you more likely to develop augmentation. Short-acting rather than extended-release (ER) or longer-acting dopamine drugs (i.e., pramipexole vs pramipexole ER) are considered by many RLS providers to increase your chances of augmentation. One of the reasons that carbidopa/levodopa fell out of favor compared to the three dopamine agonists is because it causes even higher rates of augmentation. Iron deficiency might also place you at higher risk, but iron deficiency should be corrected prior to taking dopamine medications, so this risk can be mitigated. The longer you take the medications and the higher the dose you take, the more likely it is that you will develop augmentation. This is why doses of dopamine agonists should be kept low. Finally, if you have taken dopamine agonists in the past and developed augmentation at that time, you're at greater risk of having augmentation again if you restart them.

It can be very frustrating for people to hear, but oftentimes the reason they're suffering so much from their RLS is because of the medication they are taking that is supposed to be helping. Augmentation is one of the most common reasons that someone with RLS will transition from being cared for by primary care to being seen in a specialty clinic. The good news is that once you stop the dopamine agonist, your RLS should go back to being no worse than it was before you started the medication; augmentation is reversible.

To understand why augmentation occurs, we must circle back to the neuroscience of RLS. When you take a dopamine agonist (or carbidopa/levodopa), you are stimulating the dopamine receptors in the brain. This has two effects: improving your RLS and reducing your brain's production of its own dopamine. The symptom improvement comes first, but once your brain reduces the amount of dopamine that it makes, you start to feel worse again. You become dependent on the pills to replace the effect of the dopamine you're no longer making. This will make you want to start taking the pills earlier and earlier during the day. The pills won't last all day, though, so you might start taking the pills multiple times per day. Each time you increase your dose, you further suppress your brain's own dopamine, giving you temporary relief and long-term problems. It's a vicious cycle, and one that you can never win by taking more medication.

Nils's neurologist explains to Nils that the pramipexole is likely responsible for this change in his behavior and that they need to work together to get him off it. She instructs him to start by reducing his dose to 0.5 mg and provides him a list of alternative therapies he can try instead.

Discontinuation and withdrawal

At this point, if you're already taking a dopamine agonist, you might be feeling scared, frustrated, or angry. Maybe you were not told about augmentation or ICDs when you were first started on the medications. My greatest motivation for writing this book was to empower people with RLS with this knowledge to help avoid these terrible outcomes. If you think that you have augmentation or an ICD, talk to your provider. Do not just stop the medication cold turkey. Abruptly stopping a dopamine agonist can be an absolutely miserable experience.

It is important to wean off a dopamine agonist. The higher the dose and the longer you've been taking it, the slower the process of stopping it should be. The goal of going slowly is to reduce your risk of developing **dopamine agonist withdrawal syndrome (DAWS)**. DAWS occurs when your brain can't keep up with the missing dopamine effects that it was getting from the dopamine agonists you were taking. It subsides when your brain adjusts to making its own dopamine again, but unfortunately, some people never seem to fully recover and end up having to go back to taking low-dose dopamine agonists indefinitely to prevent these withdrawal symptoms.

DAWS symptoms can include a worsening of your RLS, terrible anxiety, depression, **fatigue**, and even diffuse body pain and **low blood pressure** when you stand up. You might have your first-ever panic attack or feel like you don't even want to leave the house. You will probably have a strong desire to take the medication again. If you're thinking that this sounds like a drug addiction, you're right; the body has developed a dependence on the medication. It can take months to years for the symptoms to resolve. The only known way to treat this is to restart the dopamine agonist, but doing so will only delay the benefits you would receive from being off the drug altogether. If the symptoms of withdrawal are intolerable, though, maintaining you on a low dose is a reasonable approach that your provider might take.

It is thought that one of the biggest predictors for DAWS is the presence of an ICD. Of course, the presence of an ICD is one of the primary reasons to quickly stop a dopamine agonist, so patients can be caught between a rock and a hard place. A compromise is getting the dose down as low as possible without completely stopping the drug, which could stop the ICD while preventing withdrawal. Ideally, the dopamine agonist would be stopped eventually after the body has had a chance to adjust to the lower dose for a longer period of time.

Stopping a dopamine agonist can be difficult even if you don't go into full-blown DAWS. At the very least, going down on the medication tends to make your RLS worse. Thankfully, this type of exacerbation tends to last only about 2 weeks. There are two schools of thought on how to handle discontinuing a dopamine agonist. One strategy is to quickly wean down, suffer for 2 weeks, and force your brain to rapidly ramp up its own dopamine. This is both effective and very difficult because those 2 weeks of uncontrolled RLS can be miserable, and anyone taking this approach should be prepared for some really bad nights. Two weeks can feel like an exceedingly long time when you're suffering like this. But the suffering is finite, and people do end up feeling a lot better than they did when they were dealing with augmentation. Think of this as ripping the Band-Aid off.

The alternative approach is slower and involves transitioning onto an alternative RLS medication first before reducing the dose of the dopamine agonist. It can take a while to find an effective alternative, though, so if the reason to stop the dopamine agonist is an ICD, you might not want to spend the time going through the trial-and-error period of finding an alternative before reducing your dose. Patients who opt for this approach will still have some discomfort as they lower their dopamine agonist dose, but hopefully less so than with the first approach.

The alternative drug might not be as effective or may cause more side effects than the dopamine agonist, which further complicates the matter. Advocates for the first approach point out that once you recover from being on a dopamine agonist, you might need a much lower dose or possibly no additional medication for your RLS, which you wouldn't know if you followed the second approach and were already taking another drug. There are pros and cons of both strategies, which is why it is important to discuss these with your provider to choose the one that's best for you. Whichever way you go, your provider will be there to help you through the process. It's difficult, but you can do it, and it'll be well worth it in the end.

After dropping his dose of pramipexole to 0.5 mg nightly, Nils is able to stop his compulsive gambling. His RLS is worse, but it is manageable with the new medication prescribed by his neurologist. He gradually weans off the rest of the pramipexole over the course of 2 months. By the time he sees his neurologist again a month later, he is not having any daytime symptoms of RLS anymore, and the new medication is highly effective at treating his nighttime symptoms.

CHAPTER 8

Gabapentinoids for RLS

In this chapter, you will learn:

- Which medications are considered gabapentinoids
- How gabapentinoids are used to treat RLS
- What are common side effects of gabapentinoids
- How to discontinue gabapentinoids

Introduction

In the last chapter, you learned about dopamine agonists and how they are both highly effective and a bit scary for the possible side effects they can cause. This chapter will cover another commonly used class of medications for RLS, **gabapentinoids**. These medications can also be highly effective, but they come with a different set of risks. Over time, gabapentinoids have been replacing dopamine agonists as first-line therapy for RLS.

History

Gabapentinoids are one of the most prescribed classes of drug in the United States. The class is named after its first member, **gabapentin**, which was initially approved by the US Food and Drug Administration (FDA) in 1993 and sold as Neurontin. The FDA has only approved gabapentin for treatment of pain related to **shingles** outbreaks and for prevention of seizures in people with **epilepsy**. However, gabapentin is more commonly used to treat a wide range of other conditions, such as peripheral neuropathy pain, **migraine**, insomnia, and, of course, RLS.

In addition to the original, there are two other forms of gabapentin on the market. In 2011, **gabapentin enacarbil (Horizant)** was approved, and unlike the original gabapentin, it has an FDA indication for the treatment of RLS. An extended-release form of gabapentin is sold under the brand name Gralise, but this is not commonly prescribed for RLS as it is costlier without providing significant advantages over regular gabapentin.

The only other gabapentinoid on the market is **pregabalin**, originally marketed as Lyrica, which was approved in 2004. Like gabapentin, pregabalin is an antiseizure drug that has been used for many other purposes. Pregabalin has FDA indications for treating **seizures**, nerve pain due to spinal cord injury, peripheral neuropathy pain from **diabetes**, **fibromyalgia**, and post-shingles pain. While not approved for RLS treatment, it is frequently used for that purpose as well. Table 8.1 lists the gabapentinoids sold in the US.

The first use of gabapentin to treat RLS was reported in 1995, shortly after it hit the market. Many reports and clinical trials followed in the second half of the 1990s, which led to wider adoption of this drug as a treatment strategy. With gabapentin already recognized

TABLE 8.1 **Gabapentinoids for RLS**

Generic name	Brand name	Generic available
Gabapentin	Neurontin	Yes
Gabapentin enacarbil*	Horizant	No
Pregabalin	Lyrica	Yes

*Gabapentin enacarbil is the only FDA-approved gabapentinoid for RLS.

as a potential treatment for RLS, it did not take long for studies of pregabalin to follow once it entered the market. These studies, performed in the late 2000s, had positive results, and they confirmed that gabapentinoids are, on the whole, effective for treating RLS. This was particularly timely research, as this was around when researchers were recognizing impulse control disorders as a complication of dopamine agonists, the other prominent class of medications for RLS (see Chapter 7). Having an alternative to dopamine agonists was very important.

When gabapentinoids were first being developed, they were expected to work like **GABA (gamma-aminobutyric acid)**, which is how they got their name. The idea had been to find a drug that controlled seizures like other GABA medications did. Although chemically gabapentin might look like GABA, it turned out that gabapentin is not actually a GABA drug at all; it doesn't work by binding to GABA receptors or affecting GABA activity. Nevertheless, the name stuck.

How gabapentin and pregabalin actually work is not well understood. There is some evidence that gabapentinoids might reduce glutamate activity, which would make sense in the context of RLS where there is excessive glutamate activity. The drugs are known to bind to receptors called **alpha-2-delta receptors**, but how that leads to all of the clinical benefits seen with these drugs is uncertain. This property of the drugs gave them their other name: **alpha-2-delta ligands**. The terms "gabapentinoids" and "alpha-2-delta ligands" are interchangeable.

Sonya is a 58-year-old woman who is seeing her primary care doctor for ongoing management of her RLS. At her last visit, she started taking iron supplements at her doctor's suggestion. Now, 3 months later, she reports that she is only about 10% better, and she would like more to be done about her legs. After reviewing the potential side effects, Sonya's doctor starts her on gabapentin 300 mg every evening.

Sonya's story is very common, as gabapentin is often the first medication selected when starting prescription drug treatment for RLS. An alternative approach would have been to start the iron pills and gabapentin at the same time, providing relief for the RLS while the iron supplements gradually increased her iron levels. If the iron were effective, she could then stop the gabapentin. The decision on whether or not to try iron first or try it in conjunction with a prescription drug depends on how severe the symptoms are. If you can't tolerate waiting months for iron to help, you can ask your provider for a prescription medication, such as gabapentin, to help in the meantime.

Dosing

Gabapentin

Gabapentin is a unique drug in that the range of doses that are prescribed is quite large, and the response patients have to these doses is highly variable. The variability in gabapentin dosing comes from differences in how people absorb the drug. Simply put, some people just don't absorb it well. You might take 100 mg and find the side effects to be overwhelming, while someone else might take 1200 mg and feel nothing from it. There is a lot of trial and error involved in getting your dose right. A usual starting point is 300 mg in the evening. If you don't feel any impact of this dose, though, your provider can guide you through rapidly increasing the dose until you feel the effects. If the effects are positive, then you are on the right dose. If the effects are unpleasant and you haven't noticed any benefits, this is not the right drug for you.

If you have symptoms throughout the day, gabapentin can be taken up to three times per day, and it is usually fine to stack the doses close together (e.g., afternoon, dinner, and bedtime) rather than spreading them out evenly throughout the day. The body usually can't absorb more than 600 mg at a time, so if you need a higher dose than that, it's best to split the doses. It is more effective to take 600 mg after dinner and 600 mg at bedtime than to take all 1200 mg after dinner. It is also acceptable to use these medications on an as-needed basis. Maybe you need 300 mg nightly with an additional 300 mg only before a long flight. Your provider can tailor your prescription accordingly.

Gabapentin enacarbil

Gabapentin enacarbil is specifically designed to be better absorbed in the intestines than gabapentin; thus, more of the active gabapentin gets to the bloodstream. If you tried gabapentin and it didn't work for you, gabapentin enacarbil might still be worth trying because you'll probably absorb it better and your blood levels of gabapentin will be higher than they were when you were taking original gabapentin. Gabapentin enacarbil also has the advantage of being longer acting, meaning it only needs to be taken once in the evening. The primary negative to gabapentin enacarbil vs traditional gabapentin is cost. Even if it is covered by your insurance, you might have a much higher copay for it than for gabapentin.

Pregabalin

Pregabalin is absorbed by the intestines more readily than gabapentin, and the dosing range is smaller with more predictable responses. Fewer people report that taking pregabalin is imperceptible, though the effect they feel might be positive or negative. Your provider will probably start you on 50 or 75 mg in the evening. The maximum evening dose is 300 mg. Some people will take it more than once per day, in which case the maximum dose is 600 mg divided into two 300 mg or three 200 mg doses. Table 8.2 summarizes the doses used for each of the gabapentinoids.

It is very important to note that if you have kidney disease, your doses of gabapentinoids must be adjusted. While gabapentinoids do not damage your kidneys, they are cleared from the blood by the kidneys, so if you have kidney disease, the drugs can build up and

TABLE 8.2 **Common doses of gabapentinoids for patients
with normal kidney function**

Generic name	Starting dose	Dose adjustments	Maximum recommended dose*
Gabapentin	300 mg nightly	300 mg as tolerated	1200 mg per night, 3600 mg per 24 hours
Gabapentin enacarbil	600 mg at dinnertime	None	600 mg at dinnertime
Pregabalin	50-75 mg nightly	50-75 mg as tolerated	300 mg per night, 600 mg per 24 hours

* People with kidney disease have lower maximum dose recommendations.

cause serious side effects. Your prescribing provider will need to scale back your dose according to your degree of kidney disease. Although gabapentin enacarbil is not recommended for patients undergoing dialysis treatments, both gabapentin and pregabalin can be used in this setting as long as your dose is kept low.

> Sonya calls her doctor a week after her last visit. The gabapentin is doing nothing to help her legs. Her doctor recommends doubling the dose to 600 mg, but this is still no help. Another week goes by and Sonya seeks further advice. She is told to increase to 900 mg. When 900 mg is equally ineffective, Sonya's doctor recommends trying gabapentin enacarbil 600 mg instead.

It seems Sonya is among the sizable percentage of people who feel no effect from gabapentin. In this case, trying gabapentin enacarbil or pregabalin would both be great second choices. Often, the decision on which drug you try next is determined by your insurance coverage. Pregabalin, as a generic medication, tends to be cheaper, but gabapentin enacarbil is the one that is FDA approved for RLS. Medically, both are reasonable to try, though, so you and your provider can choose either option next based on which one you can get covered.

Side effects

Gabapentinoids are among the safest medications on the market. An overdose of acetaminophen or aspirin is far more likely to be fatal than an overdose of gabapentin (not that I recommend it, of course). The people most prone to serious side effects from gabapentinoids are those with kidney disease who have not had their doses adjusted to account for their kidney function, causing a buildup of medication in the blood. The classic symptoms of gabapentinoid **toxicity** are the combination of muscle jerks (i.e., myoclonus) and loss of muscle tone (the medical term is **asterixis**). For example, you might be holding still and suddenly jerk or you are holding your arm out and it suddenly collapses. Either of these—muscle jerks or muscle collapse—can be seen in other conditions individually, but if you have them both at the same time, it is a red flag for excessive gabapentinoid levels.

It's very unlikely that anyone with normally functioning kidneys will develop toxicity unless they intentionally (or unintentionally) overdose. However, gabapentinoids can also cause plenty of other side effects in anyone, even those with full kidney function. First off, they can lead to significant sedation and confusion. This is more likely to happen in older adults, but even young adults who are particularly sensitive to them can experience this. They can also impair memory, cause blurry vision, and impair coordination. If you are taking the drug multiple times per day, the sedation might interfere with your ability to function, but most people taking it only at night do well with it. You might actually like the fact that these medications can be sedating as they could help you sleep better at night.

Gabapentinoids can also induce weight gain. This might be enough of a reason not to take a gabapentinoid, particularly compared to the dopamine agonists (Chapter 7), which are weight neutral (unless you develop an eating impulse control disorder). Thankfully, weight gain is not a terribly common side effect of these drugs, so if your provider suggests it, you might decide to try one and just monitor your weight.

More common is swelling in the legs, called **peripheral edema**. This can be distressing but isn't usually dangerous. There is no need to take fluid pills (**diuretics**) to try to get rid of this fluid because that can lead to kidney damage. If you get mild peripheral edema from gabapentinoids, it's best to ignore it, and if it's substantial peripheral edema, you probably want to find an alternative medication; diuretics are not the way to go. Generally speaking, it's best not to try to counteract the side effects of one drug by taking another drug if you can avoid it.

Although uncommon, gabapentinoids can exacerbate depression or even trigger it in people who have never had depression before. In the most severe cases, the side effect of depression can reach the point of suicidal thoughts and behaviors if the drug is not stopped. If you experience any mood changes while taking a gabapentinoid, be sure to let your provider know right away. Thankfully, this side effect is rare enough that these medications are still used regularly in patients with a history of depression. You do not need to avoid this class of drugs just because you have had trouble with depression in the past, but you do need to know that this risk exists so that you can report it to your provider if you observe your mood changing when you start it.

Sonya tries gabapentin enacarbil for 2 weeks before calling back to her doctor to report that she feels groggy and "drugged up" from this medication. She doesn't like taking it, but it is at least helping her legs and she is sleeping better since starting it. The daytime hangover she is getting is not worth the benefits, though. She asks for an alternative. Her doctor prescribes pregabalin 50 mg in the evening.

Even though she didn't feel anything from gabapentin, Sonya experiences one of the more common side effects from gabapentin enacarbil because she is absorbing it better than she did gabapentin. As expected, it's helping her legs, but with these side effects, a change has to be made. Despite their similarity, the sedation from gabapentin or gabapentin enacarbil does not always translate to sedation from pregabalin. Some people tolerate one much better than they tolerate the others, so switching between them makes sense. It is common for patients to try all three gabapentinoids to choose the one that works best without side effects.

Complications

Both gabapentin and pregabalin have been reported as potential causes of liver disease, but these are only sporadic case reports, and the risk for this is extremely low. In general, these medications do not damage the heart, lungs, kidney, liver, or other organs. Another benefit of gabapentinoids is their lack of interaction with other medications. They can be safely combined with almost all other drugs with one big caveat: they enhance the sedative effects of other sedating drugs. Thus, if you were to take a gabapentinoid with an opioid painkiller (e.g., oxycodone), for example, your risk of overdosing from the opioid goes up. While these medications are routinely combined in practice, this must be done cautiously.

Gabapentinoids do not cause augmentation. You can stay on one indefinitely and not risk your RLS symptoms getting worse, as is so often the case with dopamine agonists. It's also unlikely that you would develop significant tolerance to an effective dose. Once you find the right dose, it's likely to continue working without the need to take higher doses over time. And gabapentinoids do not cause impulse control disorders. This is a complication that is very specific to dopamine agonists, so you don't have to worry about that if you are taking a gabapentinoid for your RLS. It is for all these reasons that gabapentinoids have taken over as the preferred initial medication for RLS.

Unfortunately, there is the potential for gabapentinoids to be **abused**. That means people who are prescribed one of these medications are taking more than they are prescribed or they are misusing them by combining them with other substances for the purpose of getting an enhanced high. As noted above, gabapentinoids can add to the sedative effects of other medications. This is a side effect providers try to prevent, but it's an effect some people seek out against medical advice. For this reason, pregabalin is a **controlled substance**. Despite the fact that gabapentin and pregabalin are very similar, gabapentin is not a federally controlled substance. Some states, however, list gabapentin as a controlled substance alongside pregabalin.

The US Drug Enforcement Agency (DEA) has six levels of regulation for prescription drugs: five for controlled substances, called "**schedules**," and a sixth level that contains all of the noncontrolled substances. The DEA places a drug on one of its schedules based on how much they think the drug can be abused or cause **dependence** (addiction). Schedule I drugs are always prohibited; there is no accepted medical use, and they cannot be prescribed. Schedule II is the most tightly regulated of the prescribed drugs, whereas Schedule V is less regulated due to the lower predicted abuse and dependence rates.

Pregabalin is a Schedule V medication, meaning that of all the drugs that can cause abuse or dependence, pregabalin is among the least likely to do so. Being on Schedule V means that your prescription and refills can only last for 6 months instead of 12 for noncontrolled substances, and you might need to show your driver's license to collect your prescription. It also means there are restrictions on your pharmacy transferring your prescription to another pharmacy if they are out of stock of the medication. If you don't live in a state that considers gabapentin a controlled substance, you can get a 1-year prescription, and that prescription could be transferred if needed.

> Sonya finds 50 mg of pregabalin to be insufficient, and under her doctor's guidance, she works up to 150 mg with good benefit for her legs and much fewer side effects than she had from gabapentin enacarbil. She tells her doctor that she is getting a little swelling in her ankles, but it is a fair trade to get relief from her RLS. She worries, though, because she isn't sure she should stay on this long term because she heard that it can be difficult to stop or cause long-term harm to her body.

Sonya's concerns are common and understandable. Thankfully, there is scant evidence that gabapentinoids cause long-term harm. They have been on the market for decades, and some people have been taking them for that long. It's certainly possible that a long-term risk will be discovered some day, but for now, this is not a significant concern. While it's true that if you have taken a gabapentinoid for many years it could be somewhat difficult to stop, even this risk is relatively low.

Discontinuation and withdrawal

Discontinuing a gabapentinoid is markedly easier than stopping a dopamine agonist that you've been taking for a long time. Unlike the miserable experience of dopamine agonist withdrawal, few people report major problems when they stop gabapentinoids. If you're on a low dose, such as 300 to 600 mg of gabapentin or 75 to 150 mg of pregabalin, you will likely be able to stop cold turkey with no trouble, but you should discuss this with your provider before doing so. If you are on a higher dose, it's best to wean down, but your provider can wean you down quickly. Since gabapentinoids have antiseizure properties, there is concern that abrupt discontinuation of a high dose could trigger a seizure.

More likely, though, for patients without a seizure disorder, withdrawal from a gabapentinoid—if you experience any symptoms at all—would take the form of anxiety or agitation, heart palpitations, and sweating. Withdrawal symptoms go away if you restart some gabapentin and wean off more slowly. Given the rarity of developing gabapentinoid dependence and the relative ease with which most patients can stop them, this tends not to be a barrier to their use. On the whole, gabapentinoids are considered the safest class of medication for RLS.

CHAPTER 9

Opioids for RLS

In this chapter, you will learn:

- Which medications are considered opioids
- How opioids are used to treat RLS
- What are common side effects of opioids
- What are the dangers of opioids
- How to discontinue taking opioids

Introduction

If dopamine agonists and gabapentinoids have not worked well for you for one reason or another, your provider might talk to you about opioids. This chapter will review the range of medications that are considered opioids. It will cover what you should expect if you are going to start opioid therapy, including the rules and the dangers, and also give you tips for how to stop these medications.

History

There are written accounts of **opium**, a naturally occurring, mind-altering and pain-relieving substance that comes from the seeds of opium poppies, being used by people suffering from RLS for at least 200 years. Given that opium use dates back thousands of years to before the common era, it has almost certainly been used for a lot longer than that. Opium and its naturally occurring derivatives morphine and codeine are collectively referred to as **opiates**. Opioids, by contrast, are medications that have been synthesized to resemble the properties of opium. Many medications are considered opioids, including hydrocodone, oxycodone, hydromorphone, methadone, tramadol, fentanyl, and buprenorphine.

It is common to hear opiates and opioids referred to interchangeably with either term, but technically, opiates are natural and opioids are synthetic, either partially (chemically derived from an opiate) or entirely (no opiates are used in synthesis). Another common term for this entire group of drugs is **narcotics**, but that term has legal connotations, so for this chapter, "opioids" will be used as a generic term for all natural and synthetic opium-related products.

The modern era for research on the use of opioids for RLS began in the 1980s as clinicians began publishing reports of successful use of opioid treatments for their patients. By the 1990s, clinical trials of tramadol, oxycodone, and propoxyphene (an opioid that was removed from the US market in 2010) found that all of these medications could be beneficial for RLS, although in reality, many RLS experts were already aware of the treatment potential of opioids by the time the formal research was published. In the 2000s, additional medications, including methadone, were studied, again with positive results. With multiple different opioids demonstrating benefits for RLS, the conclusion was that opioids, as a drug class, are highly effective treatments.

Opioid drugs bind to opioid receptors. Opioid receptors exist in the brain, spinal cord, and nerves, which means their impact can be widespread in the body. All of the opioids that are commonly used for RLS bind to the mu-opioid receptor. "Mu" is the Greek letter for "m" that was assigned to this receptor because the receptor is sensitive to morphine. Why and how opioids are so effective for RLS is not well understood. Most likely, there is an interaction between the brain's dopamine and opioid systems, but much more research needs to be done to fully understand this relationship.

Although certain opioids come in special formulations and are sold as brand-name drugs, all opioids used in RLS can be obtained in generic form. None of them, however, are US Food and Drug Administration approved for RLS. Opioids are classified as Schedule II drugs, meaning they have a high abuse and dependence risk, with the exceptions of buprenorphine (Schedule III) and tramadol (Schedule IV).

The risk of dependence with opioid drugs is well known. You have likely either known someone or at least heard on the news about someone who has died of an overdose after developing opioid use disorder (OUD), the medical term used to describe a problematic use of opioids that leads to harm or distress to the patient. As you read this chapter, it is important to remember that opioids are dangerous drugs with potentially fatal consequences. Nevertheless, they play a critical role in the treatment of RLS and have been positively life-changing for those who need them.

> Jack is a 71-year-old man who has been treated for RLS for the past year. In that time, he has cut out caffeine and alcohol, received an iron infusion, started a daily exercise routine, and tried both gabapentin and pregabalin with intolerable side effects from both. He is currently on pramipexole 0.5 mg nightly and tells his sleep doctor that it is no longer helping. He is miserable. RLS is ruining his retirement because he can't travel or even sit through a movie with his spouse.

Jack has **refractory** RLS, meaning that his RLS is not adequately treated despite having tried the first-line treatments (iron, gabapentinoids, and dopamine agonists). Given the severity of his symptoms, it is reasonable for Jack's doctor to consider starting him on an opioid. Before doing so, though, Jack will need to be screened for his potential to develop an addiction to opioids. If you are in this position, your provider will likely use a questionnaire, such as the **Opioid Risk Tool** (see appendix), to help predict your risk of becoming dependent on opioids. While these types of screening questionnaires are far from perfect, if your risk of developing dependence is high, you might consider alternative therapies first or your provider might keep an extra close watch on your use of the drug and behavior while taking it. A low score does not mean that opioids are completely safe for you, but it does provide some reassurance.

Thankfully, the risk of developing opioid use disorder from the opioids prescribed for RLS seems to be lower than the risk when used for other purposes, such as chronic pain. When used for pain, escalating doses of opioids are often needed, but fortunately, that is not typically the case in RLS. Effective doses of opioids for RLS tend to be much lower than for chronic pain, and once an effective dose is reached, you can usually maintain that dose indefinitely.

Each clinic will have its own rules for managing patients on chronic opioid therapy in order to keep them as safe as possible. After a conversation about the risks and benefits of initiating opioid therapy, you might be asked to sign a contract with the prescriber detailing certain rules you will be expected to follow. Common rules include not getting refills early (including if you lose your pills); not obtaining other controlled substance prescriptions from other providers without notifying your opioid prescriber first; not mixing your prescribed opioid with alcohol, illicit drugs, or other sedating medications; keeping your prescription safe from theft; and not sharing your medication with anyone else. Opioid contracts are not punishments and do not reflect any personal judgments about you or your risk of abusing opioids; they're safety measures and tools to improve communication between you and your clinician.

Another common requirement is that you might be asked to agree in advance to randomly timed urine drug testing. This is done for two purposes. First, your prescriber needs to make sure that you haven't been combining the prescribed opioid with other drugs that could create a fatal overdose. Second, your prescriber needs to make sure that you are actually taking the drug that is prescribed. A urine drug screen that shows no use of the prescribed drug is as concerning as one that shows the use of multiple drugs, as it raises the possibility of **diversion**, meaning the drug is being given or sold to someone to whom it was not prescribed. Like contracts, urine drug testing is not done as a punishment, and it does not reflect your provider's personal opinion of you or your behavior. But with tens of thousands of people dying every year from opioids, these drugs must be carefully monitored to reduce risks.

Dosing and prescribing of opioids

There are a few general principles providers use with opioids for RLS. First, "start low and go slow." This means that you will be started on as low a dose as possible, and the dosage will be raised very cautiously.

TABLE 9.1 Common dosing of opioids for patients with RLS

Generic name	Starting dose	Dose adjustments (every 4–7 days until effective)	Maximum recommended dose per day (can be divided into multiple smaller doses if immediate release)
Buprenorphine	0.3–0.5 mg per evening	0.3–0.5 mg	6 mg
Codeine	15–30 mg per evening	30 mg	180 mg
Hydrocodone	5 mg	5 mg	45 mg
Methadone	2.5 mg 3 hours before bedtime	2.5–5 mg	20 mg
Morphine	10 mg per evening	10 mg	45 mg
Oxycodone	5 mg	5 mg	30 mg
Tramadol	50 mg	50 mg	200 mg

Reproduced and modified with permission of Elsevier from Silber et al. in *Mayo Clinic Proceedings*, volume 96, issue 7, July 2021.

Table 9.1 provides common dosing for the opioids most often used for RLS. Since very few studies have been done to figure out the optimal dosing of opioids for RLS, these numbers come mostly from expert opinion, such as the report by the Medical Advisory Board of the Restless Legs Syndrome Foundation (see appendix). Unlike dopamine agonists, patients seldom need the maximum dosages of opioids, and it's more likely that you would end up on the lowest dose than ever hit the recommended maximum dose. The goal is to take as little opioid as is absolutely necessary to treat your symptoms, even if that means you still have mild residual symptoms. The goal isn't always to eliminate your symptoms; the real goal is to improve your quality of life, which can often be achieved without 100% reduction of your RLS.

The second principle is that if one opioid either does not work well or causes side effects, then another should be tried. Each opioid is different enough that one failure doesn't predict another failure. Essentially, you and your provider can work through each of these options until you find the one that works best for you. Among the list of opioids used for RLS, methadone is thought to be the most likely to work. While methadone might cause intolerable side effects (which will be discussed later in this chapter), the success rate, if you tolerate it, is very high.

Buprenorphine is gaining more and more popularity over time and is another good choice. Tramadol, with its lower abuse and dependence rating (Schedule IV), is often tried first, but it is less likely to be as effective as methadone. And while there is a theoretical potential for tramadol to induce augmentation, this is a much lower risk than with dopamine agonists. None of the other opioids cause augmentation, so this is unique to tramadol.

Oxycodone and hydrocodone were more widely prescribed in the past, but current trends favor methadone and buprenorphine due to concerns about addiction; methadone and buprenorphine are thought to cause less dependence than oxycodone and hydrocodone. Codeine is lower **potency**, meaning it takes a lot more of the drug to get an effect, than the other opioids, and the success rate with codeine is relatively low compared to the others. Morphine tends to be used infrequently. Morphine tends to cause more side effects than some of the others and is probably the least often prescribed for RLS among the opioids.

Third, longer-acting medications are preferred to shorter-acting medications. RLS often starts in the evening before bed, and the medication needs to work for up to 10 hours or more to adequately treat the condition without you waking up in the middle of the night with **rebound** RLS. That means for the shorter-acting drugs such as oxycodone and morphine, the extended-release forms are usually preferred, though there is a place for shorter-acting drugs for patients with a relatively shorter duration of symptoms.

The length of time a drug is active in your body is related to its **half-life**. A half-life is how long it takes half of a drug to be processed in the body. After one half-life, 50% of a drug is gone. After two half-lives, 75% is gone, and after three half-lives, 87.5% is gone, and so forth. Table 9.2 includes the half-lives of the commonly prescribed opioids. Not everybody processes drugs at the same speed, so half-lives are reported with a range to reflect the possible rates at which any particular person might clear the drug. The half-life numbers do not account for any interactions with other drugs you might be taking

TABLE 9.2 Common opioids for RLS and their duration of action

Generic name	Half-life	Duration	Extended-release availability
Buprenorphine	20–44 hours	Long	Yes, but not used for RLS
Codeine	2.5–4 hours	Short	No
Hydrocodone	7–9 hours	Medium	Yes
Methadone	8–59 hours	Long	No
Morphine	2–4 hours	Short	Yes
Oxycodone	3.5–4 hours	Short	Yes
Tramadol	6.3–7.9 hours	Medium	Yes

that could increase or decrease the time it takes for the body to eliminate the drug.

Like the dopamine agonists and gabapentinoids, opioids can be used on an as-needed basis under the guidance of your provider. One possible method is to use a gabapentinoid nightly and add an opioid just on the nights your legs are especially restless. There are many strategies for using opioids, and they do not all require daily use.

Many of the opioids are more readily available as combination pills with other medications. For example, hydrocodone is usually cheaper when sold as hydrocodone/acetaminophen than when sold as pure hydrocodone. Codeine is also frequently combined with other medications, particularly acetaminophen. The opioids will typically work just as well even when given as a combination pill, but you have to be conscious of the fact that you're taking two medications even if they come as one pill.

Buprenorphine is available both as a stand-alone medication and as a combination with the drug naloxone. This combination is commonly known by the brand name Suboxone. Like other combination medications, buprenorphine/naloxone can treat RLS, but the buprenorphine is the effective component. Buprenorphine/naloxone has been uniquely regulated by the Drug Enforcement Agency, making it especially difficult to prescribe without additional training and licensure. This has prevented its widespread adoption as an RLS medication, but these rules have been changed recently, and it is becoming easier for any prescriber to offer this therapy to patients with RLS.

Jack's doctor performs an opioid risk assessment and Jack is deemed low risk for opioid use disorder. His doctor recommends that Jack start methadone therapy for his RLS. He tells Jack that this would probably be the best way to quickly restore his quality of life. He recommends starting with half of a 5 mg pill and instructs Jack to take it 3 hours

(Continued)

(Continued)

before bedtime. He also recommends that Jack start cutting his 0.5 mg pramipexole in half with the goal of weaning off this entirely. Jack tells his doctor that getting relief from his RLS sounds fantastic, but he's scared of opioids in general and wants to know more about the side effects before agreeing to start one.

Side effects

There are many side effects associated with opioids. One of the most famous is constipation. Constipation is such a problem from opioids that other medications are made just to counteract this side effect. This is why opioids are also sold as antidiarrhea agents. Unless you have other reasons for constipation, many people on low doses of opiates for RLS can handle the side effect of constipation by taking over-the-counter supplements, such as polyethylene glycol (marketed as MiraLAX). If you have severe RLS and get substantial relief from opioids, this is a tradeoff you might be willing to make. While some of the other side effects of opioids might wear off in time as you adjust to the medication, constipation usually doesn't. Unfortunately, if you have significant constipation from an opioid, it's likely to remain a problem as long as you're on that drug.

Other digestive side effects include nausea and vomiting. If this happens, you'll probably want to switch opioids. You will not necessarily have this side effect from all opioids. If the reaction occurred due to a natural opiate, try a synthetic opioid instead next time.

Opioids can also be highly sedating. Unlike constipation, this effect usually wears off reasonably soon after you start therapy, except for methadone, which is associated with persistent sleepiness in some people. At the low doses used for RLS, you might never experience sedation. Some people might experience dizziness from these drugs, which is another side effect that could wear off in time. Myoclonus—sporadic muscle jerks—are another possible side effect, but this is less common.

Some of the opioids have idiosyncratic side effects that you would only expect from that particular drug, not from the whole class of opioids. For example, buprenorphine might cause trouble sleeping rather than sleepiness. It can also trigger significant anxiety or panic. And most prescriptions for buprenorphine are in the form of strips placed under the tongue or inside the cheek, and people who use these are at increased risk of dental cavities, particularly if they brush their teeth directly after taking the medication. If you use buprenorphine strips, the recommendation to protect your teeth is to swish and swallow water after taking the medication, wait an hour before brushing your teeth, and get regular dental checkups.

Methadone is unique in that it can trigger daytime sleep attacks, claustrophobia, or a sensation of "air hunger," which is the feeling that you can't catch your breath. Tramadol is the opioid most closely associated with an increased risk of seizures. If you are being prescribed an opioid, your provider will review the unique side effects associated with your specific medication.

Complications

Beyond side effects, opioids can have numerous dangerous consequences that can complicate your treatment. The number one complication to address is dependence. Opioids can cause a euphoric sensation, and the brain can start to crave more and more of these medications. It is important for anyone treated with opioids, as well as their loved ones, to be aware of the signs and symptoms of opioid use disorder. These include increasing the dose of your own medicine without consulting your provider, increasing use of the medication despite negative consequences from doing so, obtaining multiple prescriptions for opioids from different sources or buying illicitly, craving the medication, and experiencing symptoms of withdrawal from missing doses of the medication.

Withdrawal symptoms include sweating, irritability, insomnia, agitation, diarrhea, and intense cravings for the medication. If you are taking opioids already and are concerned that this might apply to you, it is important to speak to your prescriber. You can also contact the Substance Abuse and Mental Health Services Administration hotline at 1-888-662-HELP; they are open 24 hours a day, 365 days per year.

The primary danger of opioid use disorder is that you could escalate the amount you are taking to an unsafe level, causing a fatal overdose. Opioids can be fatal because they cause **respiratory depression**. This means that your brain slows down your breathing and makes your breathing shallow and ineffective. The combination of sedation and inadequate breathing leads to an increase in carbon dioxide in the blood combined with not enough oxygen getting to your heart, which then stops beating.

Not all opioid-related deaths are due to respiratory depression, though. Some opioids can change the way your heart conducts electricity, which means that they can directly stop your heart from beating. People with a condition called **long QT syndrome** or who take medications that cause a long **QT interval** should be cautious when adding an opioid that prolongs the QT interval even further. This condition can be assessed with a routine **electrocardiogram**.

The amount of an opioid that could be fatal depends on many factors, including how experienced your body is in processing opioids. If you have never been on more than the small amount prescribed for RLS or have recently started opioids, it will take far less to kill you than it would someone who has been on high doses for many years. The risk of overdose is also related to other substances that you might be taking, including other prescribed medications, alcohol, or illicit drugs.

The risk of dying from an overdose is reduced if someone nearby has access to the opioid reversal agent naloxone (marketed as Narcan). If you have taken too much of an opioid, a bystander can administer naloxone, a nasal spray, and reverse the effects of the opioid. Naloxone has saved thousands of lives and should be prescribed to anyone on more than minimal opioids to have on hand in case of an emergency. Most RLS patients are on minimal doses of opioids, though, so it is uncommon for patients who are on opioids exclusively for RLS to receive naloxone prescriptions. At the time of this writing, naloxone was just approved to be sold over the counter, so it will soon be available for anyone to have on hand.

Fortunately, compared to the higher doses used to treat chronic pain, the low doses of opioids used for RLS are 86% less likely to cause opioid use disorder. Less than 1% of RLS patients treated at standard RLS doses of opioids would be predicted to develop dependence. As a result, it is generally felt that the fear of opioid use disorder should not preclude opioid therapy for people with severe and refractory RLS. For most of these people, the benefits of the opioids outweigh the risks.

Two other complications of opioid therapy are worth noting as they can cause significant problems themselves: **central sleep apnea** and low **testosterone**. All opioids can cause central sleep apnea, which occurs when your brain intermittently does not signal your **diaphragm** to breathe while you're asleep. This is similar to the respiratory depression that can occur during an overdose, but not as severe. Central sleep apnea from opioids is different from the more common and well-known form of sleep apnea, obstructive sleep apnea, which is caused by a collapse of the airway while sleeping.

If you sleep alone, it would be easy for your central sleep apnea to go undetected. If you have a bedpartner, you might be told that you intermittently stop breathing in your sleep. Unlike the loud snoring that is classic in obstructive sleep apnea, central sleep apnea might be silent. If you are already treated for obstructive sleep apnea and use a **continuous positive airway pressure (CPAP) machine**, the report from the machine can alert you to the presence of central sleep apnea, which is not usually as effectively treated by CPAP as obstructive sleep apnea.

Symptoms of central sleep apnea that should prompt you to seek out further evaluation of your sleep are waking up more frequently during the night, waking up with headaches, poor concentration, and daytime sleepiness. While opioids can be sedating when you first start them, if you remain sleepy for weeks or months after starting opioids, consider central sleep apnea, rather than a drug side effect, as the reason why. Central sleep apnea is treatable, but the only way to eliminate the problem would be to stop the opioid or try a different opioid, as you might not have this complication from every opioid.

Low testosterone is a relatively common complication, particularly for men taking chronic opioids. Symptoms of low testosterone are fatigue, depression, low libido, and erectile dysfunction. As with other opioid consequences, low testosterone is more likely to occur with higher doses. Methadone and oxycodone, especially long-acting oxycodone, are among the most likely opioids to cause low testosterone.

Keep in mind, though, that just because a blood test might identify a decrease in testosterone levels does not mean you will experience the symptoms of low testosterone. For that reason, testosterone levels are not routinely checked in patients on long-term opioid therapy. However, if you are experiencing symptoms that are consistent with low testosterone, it would be reasonable to discuss this with your provider and have your levels checked.

> Jack is nervous about trying methadone, but he's been so miserable that he decides to proceed. When he returns to the clinic 2 months later, he is very excited to report that methadone has been a miracle for him. He is tolerating it well with mild constipation and no other side effects. He has stopped his pramipexole entirely and has mild residual RLS symptoms. He asks about trying the full 5 mg pill, which his doctor agrees with. At the end of the visit, Jack expressed great appreciation for his doctor's help but inquired about how much longer he would have to take the methadone.

Discontinuation and withdrawal

A common question that comes up when patients start opioids for RLS is, "Am I going to be on this forever?" The truthful—albeit dissatisfying—answer is "maybe." If you are starting opioids to help you discontinue a dopamine agonist because you have developed augmentation, then you have a reasonable chance to stop the opioid once you have adapted to being off the dopamine agonist. Likewise, if you are scheduled for an iron infusion, you might need an opioid temporarily until you start to perceive the benefits of the iron in about 2 months, at which point you might be able to stop the opioid.

However, many patients in these situations find their quality of life so much better on low-dose opioids that they have no strong desire to stop them; life is finally good! If you have sufficient iron, have tried other medications, and are still suffering, the odds are high that you will want to stay on low-dose opioids indefinitely. Given how effective opioids can be, this is a situation you might be willing to accept.

There is no special formula for stopping opioids. The dose should be reduced slowly to avoid withdrawal. Given that most people using opioids for RLS are already on low doses, there usually aren't very many lower doses available, which means that it doesn't take long to wean off them. Your provider will help guide you through this process. Whether or not the opioid is replaced with a different RLS medication will depend on the severity of your symptoms once you stop it.

In summary, opioids are a highly effective treatment for RLS. They work when other medications have failed. Although the list of potential side effects and complications is long and scary, most of these are related to dose and can be avoided by keeping the dose low, which is almost always possible when treating RLS.

While patients on chronic opioids face opioid use contracts, urine drug screening, and potential stigma from both inside and outside the health care system, the relief these drugs provide is often well worth these downsides. At the very least, if you are suffering with RLS and have tried several other therapies already, it is worth discussing opioid therapy with your health care provider. This might be the treatment you've been searching for years.

CHAPTER 10

Benzodiazepines for RLS

In this chapter, you will learn:

- Which medications are considered benzodiazepines
- How benzodiazepines are used to treat RLS
- What are common side effects of benzodiazepines
- What are the dangers of benzodiazepines
- How to discontinue taking benzodiazepines

Introduction

The previous three chapters have covered dopamine agonists, gabapentinoids, and opioids, which are, by far, the top three classes of medication currently used for RLS. One more class of drugs deserves its own discussion, though, and those are benzodiazepines. This chapter will review the history and usage of benzodiazepine medications for RLS. Safety is a primary reason these drugs are used less often now, so risks and side effects of these drugs will be reviewed, along with how to safely discontinue them under the guidance of your health care provider.

History

Benzodiazepines (commonly called "**benzos**") were invented in the 1950s and remain very frequently prescribed even 70 years later.

Drugs like diazepam, clonazepam, alprazolam, and lorazepam fall into this drug class. Benzos serve many medical purposes related to their ability to provide sedation. Unlike the misnamed gabapentinoids, benzos actually do stimulate the gamma-aminobutyric acid (GABA) receptors in the brain. GABA reduces the activity of other neurons, so stimulating these receptors has the general effect of slowing down the brain. As a result, benzos can be used to treat anxiety, **panic attacks**, seizures, and insomnia. There are many benzos on the market in the US and many others used around the world. This chapter will focus specifically on the ones that are most likely to be used for RLS in the US.

In the late 1970s and early 1980s, doctors started reporting that their patients with RLS were improving with the use of benzos, most often clonazepam. By the 1990s, before dopamine agonists took over as the dominant medication for RLS, clonazepam was considered by many to be a first-line treatment for RLS, even though there hadn't been any formal research establishing that it worked. Since trouble sleeping is a common problem for people with RLS, these drugs were thought to help with both that symptom and the restlessness: a win-win situation.

Even to this day, there has been very little research on clonazepam for RLS, and what research there is has had mixed results. Some studies indicate that it is no better than a placebo, while others indicate that it helps with sleep more than it does with leg sensations or movements. It's unlikely that there will be much more research on clonazepam for RLS because of the potential side effects and complications described later in this chapter; other drugs are safer and more effective. The lack of data supporting its use has pushed clonazepam and the other benzos down the list of medications to use for RLS.

Further complicating the situation, benzodiazepines, like opiates, are considered addictive medications, and drug dependence is a concern. Thus, when dopamine agonists were shown to be effective, they were seen as a way to get the benefit of treating RLS without the risk of dependence (it wasn't until much later that it became clear that dopamine agonists have their own problems with dependence and withdrawal). The risk of developing benzo dependence is a common reason they are much less likely to be prescribed for RLS than they were several decades ago. In fact, the Restless Legs Syndrome Foundation goes so far as to say these drugs should not be prescribed for RLS at all anymore, although the American Academy of Sleep Medicine's position is that clonazepam can be tried if other medications fail.

Dosing and prescribing of benzodiazepines

The lack of research on benzos for RLS means that there are no established dosing guidelines. The doses of benzos that are commonly used for RLS treatment are similar to the doses used for other conditions (e.g., anxiety). Table 10.1 provides common RLS doses. The primary difference among the various benzos is the half-life; some of these medications last much longer in your body than others. Of the commonly used benzos, diazepam tends to be the longest acting and alprazolam the shortest. Table 10.2 lists the half-lives of the commonly used benzos. If you are taking a short-acting benzo and it wears off too soon, you might wake up during the night with restless legs. If you are taking a long-acting benzo, you might have a medication hangover in the morning or even feel sedated the whole next day. It can be

TABLE 10.1 **Common benzodiazepines and the typical RLS doses**

Generic name	Starting dose	Dose adjustments as tolerated	Maximum recommended nightly dose
Alprazolam	0.5 mg	0.5 mg	2 mg
Clonazepam	0.5 mg per evening	0.5 mg	2 mg
Diazepam	2-5 mg	5 mg	10 mg
Lorazepam	1 mg	1 mg	4 mg

TABLE 10.2 Common benzodiazepines for RLS and their duration of action

Generic name	Half-life	Duration
Alprazolam	12-15 hours	Short
Clonazepam	20-60 hours	Long
Diazepam	36-200 hours	Long
Lorazepam	10-20 hours	Short

difficult to find a dose of a drug that works exactly as long as you want it to without wearing off too soon or hanging around too long.

While the rule with opiates is to try each one until you find one that works well for you, that is not generally true with benzos. If you didn't respond to one, you probably won't respond to the others either. Changing benzos really only changes the half-life, not how effective it will be or the side effects. Like opiates, though, the principle of "start low and go slow" still applies. Your provider will likely recommend the lowest dose that still reduces your symptoms, even if that means that you still have mild residual restlessness.

Esther is a 73-year-old, active, and generally healthy woman who came to the sleep clinic to establish care with a new physician assistant for her RLS. She has been treated for RLS since the late 1980s by a series of primary care providers. She was started on clonazepam 0.5 mg many years ago, and over time, her primary doctors have gradually increased her dose to 3 mg nightly as that is what was required to keep her RLS under control. She tells the sleep physician assistant that the clonazepam works very well for her—she has no RLS symptoms at all—but her new primary care nurse practitioner was not comfortable continuing to prescribe the clonazepam for her. "She told me I'm too old," Esther reported to the physician assistant. "Will you just prescribe it for me?" she requests. "I really don't want

(Continued)

(Continued)
to stop it because my legs will start acting up. I don't want to live like that ever again!"

Esther, the primary care nurse practitioner, and the sleep clinic physician assistant are all in a difficult situation. Esther is justifiably concerned that coming off clonazepam would mean worsening RLS. The nurse practitioner is justifiably concerned about a 73-year-old woman, even a healthy one, taking a high dose of clonazepam both now and in the future. And the sleep physician assistant needs to find a way to balance these concerns. The physician assistant begins his evaluation by inquiring about any side effects of clonazepam that Esther might be experiencing.

Side effects

The most common complaint associated with benzos is sedation. You might feel groggy or foggy headed from these drugs. Sedation is one of the goals of the medication, but if you are feeling this way during the day when you need to be awake and alert, this becomes an unpleasant side effect. Other common side effects are confusion and unsteadiness. The unsteadiness is particularly a problem for older adults who are more prone to falls. Some people might experience dizziness, slurred speech, or muscle weakness. The higher the dose, the more likely that you will have side effects.

Complications

Benzodiazepine dependence is one of the most worrisome complications of chronic use of any benzo. The calming effect that comes over you after taking one of these pills can feel really good and encourage you to take more. It doesn't take long before even the thought of not taking a benzo can provoke substantial anxiety. Usage can escalate and your friends and family might start to notice that you appear "drugged," because you're slurring words or stumbling a bit when you walk. Continued use despite the negative impact it is having on you is the definition of dependence.

If you have been taking benzodiazepines regularly, whether or not you are concerned about dependence, it is not recommended to stop them abruptly. Long-term benzo use requires you to gradually taper off them due to concerns about going into withdrawal. Withdrawal symptoms from benzos include anxiety, insomnia, panic attacks, and agitation. If the dose is high and you've been taking them for a long time, withdrawal could in rare cases even trigger hallucinations or seizures.

Another complication of benzodiazepine use is an increased risk of dementia. It is estimated that benzo use makes you 1.5 times more likely to develop dementia over time. In studies, benzos with longer half-lives increased this risk more than benzos with shorter half-lives. And the risk also went up the longer people took a benzo, particularly 3 years or more. Likewise, benzodiazepines can be particularly bad for people who already have dementia. They can induce further memory problems, balance problems, and **delirium** (a mental state characterized by confusion, disorientation, agitation, and a general lack of awareness of surroundings). While there is a role for benzos in treating many conditions, including RLS, its benefits must be weighed against irreversible consequences, such as dementia.

Benzodiazepines, like opiates, cause respiratory depression. Overdoses can slow breathing. If there are no other sedatives in the system, such as alcohol, opioids, or muscle relaxers, an overdose of benzodiazepines is not likely to be fatal because there is a limit to the degree of respiratory depression that benzos can cause. That said, many people who overdose on benzos do have other medications or illicit drugs in their bodies at the time, and that can create the setting for a fatal overdose. Short of death, benzo overdoses can cause a prolonged **coma**. The body is very vulnerable when the brain is comatose, so even if the initial benzo overdose doesn't kill you, you are not out of the woods, and death can still occur from other medical complications that might occur in this setting.

Thankfully, there is a medication that can reverse benzodiazepine overdoses called flumazenil. It is usually given by injection or nasal spray. Flumazenil blocks the benzo from binding to the GABA receptors in the brain. This can be very helpful in waking someone up who took too much of a benzo. The downside is that it can also induce benzo withdrawal symptoms in people whose brains are accustomed to having some benzo around all the time.

Esther's sleep physician assistant reviews these potential complications with Esther. Esther is visibly dismayed. "Well, if I'd known that it was going to give me dementia, I never would have started these pills!" The sleep physician assistant reassures her that an increased risk of dementia does not mean that she will ever necessarily develop dementia, but stopping the clonazepam is still the right idea. The more likely consequence of a fall and broken bone is enough justification to find something safer. As Esther has never tried any other RLS medications, the physician assistant suggests trying gabapentin, which she agrees to do. He also sets Esther up with a schedule to wean down the clonazepam slowly over the next 6 months.

Discontinuation and withdrawal

The guiding principle behind stopping a benzo for someone who has been taking one for several years or more is to take things slowly. There is no rule that fits everybody; some people would rather move quickly and get off the drugs sooner rather than later, but others would rather avoid any withdrawal symptoms by going extra slowly. You can share your preference with your provider who will be working with you through this process to establish a mutually agreeable schedule.

One common approach is to move quickly to 50% of the dose you have been on and stay there for 1 to 2 months before going down by another 50%, continuing this process until you can stop entirely. If you have developed a dependence on benzodiazepines (**benzodiazepine use disorder**) and experience cravings or **relapses** when coming off your benzo, you will likely require a more complex strategy, including addiction counseling and potentially additional medications to help you stop these medications. Please be honest with your provider if you are struggling with the taper schedule they have established with you. They are there to help and want you to succeed.

CHAPTER 11

Additional Medications for RLS

In this chapter, you will learn:

- What medications are uncommonly used for RLS and how they work
- What are common side effects of the uncommonly used RLS medications
- When an uncommonly used RLS medication might be right for you

Introduction

Thus far, you have heard about the use of iron (Chapter 5), non-pharmacological treatments (Chapter 6), and the most frequently prescribed medications (Chapters 7 to 10) for RLS. This chapter will cover less common prescription therapies that might be a viable treatment strategy for you. These medications have one thing in common: there is very little formal research on them. What we know about how they work for RLS has come from either small research studies with only a few patients or anecdotal reports.

The medications in this chapter are approved to prevent seizures, reduce high blood pressure, prevent strokes, treat depression, and reduce the frequency of headaches. RLS is an **off-label** use for these medications, which means the US Food and Drug Administration (FDA) did not approve them for this purpose. Nevertheless, they

TABLE 11.1 **Uncommonly used prescription medications for RLS**

Drug name	Primary uses	Clinical trial with placebo performed?	Dose recommendation
Bupropion	Depression	Yes	150-300 mg daily
Carbamazepine	Seizures	Yes	200 mg once or twice
	Pain		per day*
Clonidine	Blood pressure	Yes	0.1-0.3 mg nightly
Dipyridamole	Blood clot prevention	Yes	200-400 mg nightly
Lamotrigine	Seizures	No	250 mg once or twice
	Mood stabilization		per day
Levetiracetam	Seizures	No	500-1000 mg nightly
Oxcarbazepine	Seizures	No	150-300 mg once or
			twice per day
Topiramate	Seizures	No	50-100 mg once or
	Headaches		twice per day
Valproic acid	Seizures	Yes	Up to 600 mg at
			bedtime*

*Carbamazepine and valproic acid require monitoring of blood levels of the drug with dose adjustments based on results.

have the potential to be effective and, in many cases, have fewer side effects than some of the more common RLS treatments. They are also available as generics at relatively affordable prices. Table 11.1 lists these medications, along with dose ranges that your provider can consider. Formal dosing guidelines are not available due to the lack of research to establish optimal doses. Your provider can work with you to find the best dose that balances the risks and benefits.

Not all medications that have ever been studied for RLS are included here. Some of them are no longer being sold, and others are simply not safe enough to be viable options. Others are too expensive to be practical. This chapter gives you options that may be safe and affordable enough to consider for your RLS therapy.

Cardiovascular drugs

Clonidine

The blood pressure medication clonidine has been on the market since the 1960s. Since then, it has been repurposed for many different medical conditions, such as attention deficient hyperactivity disorder (ADHD), insomnia, and pain. Clonidine's primary mechanism of action is to act in the brain to reduce the chemicals that increase blood pressure by constricting **blood vessels** throughout the body. One of these chemicals is the neurotransmitter **norepinephrine**, which could be how clonidine helps RLS. We know that some drugs that increase norepinephrine can worsen RLS, so the reduction in norepinephrine may be relevant for the treatment of RLS.

The starting dose of clonidine is 0.1 mg nightly. In the largest study of clonidine for RLS (which had only 11 subjects), the average dose used was 0.5 mg and the maximum dose was 1 mg. Common side effects included dry mouth, impaired thinking, lightheadedness, and sleepiness, and these side effects tended to set in at just 0.3 to 0.4 mg per night. Another study that looked specifically at patients with chronic kidney disease and RLS showed that very low-dose clonidine (0.075 mg) was highly effective for this particular group.

Overall, clonidine has been used for RLS for many years, mostly without data to support it. It has a reasonably good safety profile, though. If you don't already have low blood pressure, you and your provider might consider clonidine for your RLS. You will need to work closely with your provider to find the right dose for you that helps your symptoms without intolerable side effects, which can be particularly challenging with clonidine. Another thing to keep in mind if you start clonidine is that this is a medication you have to stop slowly. Abruptly discontinuing clonidine can lead to a dangerous rebound spike in blood pressure.

Dipyridamole

Dipyridamole is a relatively new player on the RLS scene, though it has been on the market since the mid-1980s. For years, providers have used it with aspirin (initially marketed as a combination pill called Aggrenox) to help prevent strokes. This use is not common today as other drugs have replaced it, but it is still used as part of testing for heart disease. It took about 30 years before it was recognized as a potential RLS medication. Dipyridamole is thought to increase the effect of adenosine. As noted in Chapter 3, impaired adenosine transmission is thought to be one of the steps in the pathway to developing RLS. When adenosine's role in causing RLS was recognized, it was logical to see if a drug that increased adenosine could improve symptoms, and it did!

While the trials have been small (15 subjects in the first one and 29 in the second), dipyridamole is one of the few drugs in this chapter that has undergone more rigorous **clinical trials**. Doses between 200 and 400 mg given at 8:00 to 9:00 PM led to improvement in RLS for most of the patients in the two trials. Starting the medication at that dose would likely cause you to have a headache, so it's best to start lower and build up.

Dipyridamole doesn't work quickly, so you have to be patient. You will hopefully start to see some improvement anywhere from several weeks to a couple of months after starting treatment. In addition to headaches, other possible side effects include an increased risk of bleeding, lightheadedness when you stand up, and upset stomach or diarrhea. Most people do not experience these side effects. If you end up discontinuing dipyridamole, it's probably because it didn't help rather than because it had intolerable side effects.

Another benefit of dipyridamole is that you can take it with many of the other RLS medications. For example, if you are taking a low-dose opioid with inadequate relief of your RLS, you could consult your provider about adding dipyridamole rather than upping your opioid dose.

Dipyridamole is available as a generic, but not all insurance companies will cover it. Sometimes, it is cheaper (or easier to get approved by insurance) to take the combination pill of dipyridamole and aspirin, which is also available as a generic. From an RLS perspective, the combo pill will work just as well, but this potentially cost-saving strategy won't work for you if you are not able to tolerate aspirin.

Desiree is a 78-year-old woman with longstanding RLS. Her primary care provider ordered her an iron infusion then started her on gabapentin, but she started gaining weight and requested an alternative therapy. Next, her provider had her try pramipexole, but when she got up to 0.5 mg, she started compulsively shopping and had to stop that medication. Desiree was more frustrated than ever. Her ongoing, severe symptoms were keeping her awake night after night. Her provider suggested that she start methadone 2.5 mg. Desiree declined this therapy because she was worried about taking an opioid medication. "Isn't there anything else you can give me?" she asked her provider. At this, her primary care provider suggested dipyridamole as an alternative. She warned Desiree that she would need to be patient with the medication, as it takes weeks to start to help and might require several steps up in dosage. Desiree agreed to try dipyridamole 50 mg nightly and return in 1 month to assess how well it was working.

Antiseizure drugs

Carbamazepine

Another 1960s medication sometimes used for RLS is carbamazepine. This drug has very successfully treated seizures and nerve pain for decades. Carbamazepine is in a class of seizure medications called **sodium channel blockers**. Blocking sodium channels helps reduce seizures, but it's not clear if this or another mechanism is responsible for the RLS benefits. It's possible that carbamazepine also acts on calcium channels, which is the way gabapentin (also an antiseizure drug) is thought to improve RLS (see Chapter 8).

Carbamazepine was first studied for RLS in the early 1980s. One study from 1984 included 174 patients, which is downright huge compared to the size of the studies on the other medications in this chapter. There was a significant benefit to carbamazepine in this study. Patients received approximately 230 mg of the drug per day. The study only lasted 5 weeks, but it showed that rapid improvement in symptoms is possible. It's not known if that benefit would be sustained over time, though.

Side effects from carbamazepine include blurry vision, abnormal eye movements, confusion, agitation, diarrhea, changes in behavior or mood, abnormal movements, trouble sleeping or sleepiness, and many others. That said, most patients who take this medication will have none of these side effects. The bigger concerns about carbamazepine are its interactions with many other medications and dangerous complications involving the blood, liver, and skin. If you and your provider are considering carbamazepine, it's very important to review all of your other prescription and over-the-counter medications and supplements to avoid interactions. You even need to avoid grapefruit juice while taking carbamazepine because it might unsafely increase the level of the drug in your body.

One dangerous complication from carbamazepine is a severe skin disorder called **Stevens-Johnson syndrome**. This syndrome causes you to develop a painful rash, followed by the top layer of your skin peeling off. It is treated like a severe burn. Some people are predisposed to developing Stevens-Johnson syndrome from carbamazepine. Blood tests can help your provider determine if you need to avoid this medication based on your genetic ancestry. Historically, this has meant screening patients with ancestry from East Asia, but this strategy missed too many at-risk patients as the gene can be found in people from South and Southeast Asia as well. Essentially, if you have Asian ancestry, testing before starting this medication is worth discussing with your provider. Not being a carrier of the gene that places you at increased risk doesn't mean you're totally out of the woods, but your risk is much lower.

Two other dangerous complications are liver failure and low sodium. Routine bloodwork can monitor for these conditions. Labs before you start taking the medication can get a baseline. Then rechecking periodically can ensure that the medication isn't causing any problems. You will probably also have your blood levels of carbamazepine checked periodically. If the medication is helping, there is no blood level that would be considered too low. Your provider will want to make sure that the level isn't too high or your risk of complications and side effects will go up.

Oxcarbazepine

The FDA approved oxcarbazepine in 1999. It is closely related to carbamazepine, as the name implies. They are structurally similar, so they are used for the same purposes, but the body processes them differently, changing their risk and side effect profiles. Oxcarbazepine has less risk of Stevens-Johnson syndrome but more risk of low sodium. Oxcarbazepine causes less change in **thyroid hormone** and testosterone than carbamazepine can. There are also fewer interactions between other drugs and oxcarbazepine, though it still has plenty of them. It's also not necessary to monitor levels of oxcarbazepine in the blood as it is with carbamazepine.

Overall, there are many advantages of this newer agent. As a result, providers often choose oxcarbazepine over carbamazepine. Be aware, however, that there is virtually no data on using oxcarbazepine for RLS, and it's not guaranteed that just because carbamazepine works, oxcarbazepine will too. They're similar, not identical. If your provider recommends oxcarbazepine, it's based on the assumption that since carbamazepine helps RLS, oxcarbazepine ought to also, and it's safer.

Topiramate

The multipurpose drug topiramate has been used for RLS with mixed results since the FDA approved it for preventing seizures in 1996. This drug is probably best known for its use in migraine. It's not known exactly how topiramate works, but it has been suggested that it can block calcium channels (like gabapentinoids, Chapter 8), stimulate gamma-aminobutyric acid (GABA) receptors (like benzodiazepines, Chapter 10), and reduce glutamate (see Chapter 3), so it could be beneficial for RLS in any or all of these ways.

Unfortunately, research on topiramate for RLS is sparse even though its theoretical potential is high. One study of 20 patients reported improvement in RLS symptoms. This study showed a benefit at the low dose of 42 mg on average. By comparison, when used for seizures, the dose can be as high as 400 mg per day. On the other hand, there are several reports of patients' RLS worsening while taking topiramate. There have also been reports of topiramate inducing RLS in patients who had not previously had it.

Common side effects of topiramate include tingling in the hands, confusion, kidney stones, eye and vision problems, changes in taste, and depression. Additionally, unlike many medications, topiramate is more likely to cause weight loss rather than weight gain, which might or might not be desirable for you.

Valproic acid

Valproic acid is another of the 1960s antiseizure medications that has been repurposed for RLS. The largest study of valproic acid in RLS included 20 patients and compared valproic acid to levodopa (Chapter 7). Patients who received valproic acid reported a larger improvement in the severity of their symptoms than those who received levodopa. Unfortunately, since this study was reported in 2004, there have been no other trials of valproic acid for RLS.

The most likely reason that this drug is not used more often is that it comes with a risk of many side effects and complications. In addition to numerous interactions with other drugs that can be difficult for your provider to navigate, you might experience weight gain, tremor, or liver, kidney, or bone marrow problems. There are also reports of Stevens-Johnson syndrome with valproic acid, though less frequently than with carbamazepine. Valproic acid requires regular blood work to monitor drug levels and potential complications. Given the elevated risk to you and the extra effort it requires on the part of your provider to monitor it, valproic acid is seldom used for RLS. Still, it might be the right choice for some patients who wish to avoid other therapies, such as opioids.

Levetiracetam

One of the relatively newer (1999) and safer antiseizure drugs is levetiracetam. Its lack of liver and kidney toxicity and ease of use from a lack of required blood tests and minimal drug-drug interactions led to a rapid increase in popularity when it was released. It would be great if this medication worked for RLS for all the same reasons that it's so popular for treating seizures.

There are no studies of levetiracetam for RLS, but one report of two patients taking 1000 mg and 500 mg, respectively, indicated long-term improvement without significant side effects. The primary side effects to watch for are mood changes and irritability. While all seizure drugs run the risk of causing depression, the risk is highest with levetiracetam. Unfortunately, there's little data to guide your provider on whether or not this is truly an effective medication for RLS.

Lamotrigine

The last of the seizure drugs that we will discuss is lamotrigine, which has been on the market in the US since 2003. This is another sodium channel blocker, which is thought to reduce glutamate activity. While it carries a risk of Stevens-Johnson syndrome, your provider will start you on a low dose and increase it slowly over about 5 weeks. When started in this manner, Stevens-Johnson syndrome is very rare.

One of the best qualities of lamotrigine is that it tends to have very few side effects. While the list of possible side effects is long, the risk that you would have any of them is low. It does not require any routine blood tests. If you are over 60 years old, your provider might want to get an electrocardiogram before and after starting treatment to ensure there are no ill effects on the electrical conduction in your heart. Generally speaking, though, most people can take this medication safely and tolerate it well. The bigger question is whether it will help your RLS. The few patients who have been reported in the scientific journals did find it beneficial, but there is still very little experience with this medication for treating RLS.

Antidepressants

Bupropion

Available since the 1980s, bupropion is a unique antidepressant. While most antidepressants target serotonin, bupropion targets dopamine and norepinephrine. In theory, this sounds like it ought to be a good treatment for RLS. In practice, though, it has not played out that way. Many people who take bupropion for depression continue to have symptoms of RLS. It is likely that bupropion's effect on dopamine is simply too weak to provide much benefit for RLS. Two clinical trials have studied bupropion for RLS, and the medication did not perform well enough to be recommended. That said, if you have depression and RLS and are considering starting an antidepressant, bupropion is the one that is least likely to exacerbate your RLS. Just don't expect that it will help your RLS much.

Antiviral medications

Amantadine

Amantadine was approved as a medication for influenza in the mid-1960s, but most influenza is now resistant to it. It turns out that this drug seems to enhance dopamine transmission and reduce glutamate, which makes it a logical choice for treating RLS. There was one study of amantadine for RLS that included 21 patients. All 21 patients reported improved RLS symptoms, with only two experiencing severe enough side effects to stop the medication. Another study compared amantadine to ropinirole (Chapter 7). Although amantadine helped, ropinirole helped more and helped for longer with fewer side effects.

It is unknown if long-term amantadine use would cause augmentation. Amantadine can cause side effects ranging from drowsiness to hallucinations, and older populations are more at risk for these problems, so the drug must be used cautiously. It's not clear if this medication offers benefits that you couldn't get from other, better-studied medications.

Desiree is reaching her limit. Her RLS is still out of control after having tried clonidine, dipyridamole, and carbamazepine over the past 6 months. Nothing has helped. "OK," she tells her provider. "I'll try the methadone if that's what you think will work." After undergoing opioid risk screening, signing a contract for use, and completing a urine drug screen, Desiree's provider starts her on methadone 2.5 mg 3 hours before bedtime. Two days later, Desiree emails her provider to admit she probably should have tried this medication first because it was already working better than any RLS therapy she had ever been on in the past.

Summary

If you have tried the first several lines of therapy, such as gabapentinoids and dopamine agonists, and found them ineffective or intolerable, one of the medications discussed in this chapter might be worth a try. Some people find that these medications keep them from taking long-term opioids or benzodiazepines, which come with the risk of dependence and overdose. Your provider can help you decide which therapy to try, but the severity of your symptoms will probably dictate how long you are willing to experiment with less established therapies. If you are suffering greatly, an opioid would be the most reliable and most efficient path to relief.

CHAPTER 12

RLS in Pregnancy

In this chapter, you will learn:

- How pregnancy increases the risk of developing RLS
- What medications for RLS you can use during pregnancy
- What happens to RLS after pregnancy
- How you can treat your RLS if you are breastfeeding

Introduction

One of the most common health conditions associated with RLS is pregnancy. This chapter reviews theories why this might occur. Even more importantly, this chapter contains information on what to do about it. If you're pregnant and reading this, you're probably wondering how much longer these unpleasant feelings will last and what you can do after delivery. This chapter will cover all of that for you also.

Lisa is a 36-year-old mother of three children, ages 3, 5, and 8 years old, who is currently 26 weeks pregnant. She is seeing her *obstetrician* for a routine visit and mentions that she is starting to have trouble sleeping. Her doctor recommends an over-the-counter sleep aid, such as diphenhydramine. A week later, she emails her doctor to say that her sleep is even worse. She just can't get comfortable. "It's strange," she tells her doctor. "It feels like I have to keep moving my legs around to get comfortable whenever I get into bed."

RLS during pregnancy

RLS can make sleep difficult during pregnancy. That will seem like an enormous understatement if you have experienced the discomfort of severe pregnancy-related ("**gestational**") RLS. Unfortunately, gestational RLS is common. It accompanies up to a quarter of all pregnancies, and it tends to be most problematic in the **third trimester**. The majority of people who experience RLS during pregnancy did not have it prior to pregnancy. And each pregnancy increases your risk of RLS. The greater the number of pregnancies, the greater the chance for RLS. So just because you didn't have RLS with your first pregnancy doesn't mean you won't get it if you get pregnant again. Whether you're starting pregnancy with pre-existing RLS or have never had it before, there's a chance of RLS with any pregnancy.

There are several theories for why RLS is so strongly tied to pregnancy. The first is related to iron. The amount of iron you need goes up during pregnancy, so iron deficiency is common. As you learned in Chapter 3, a low iron level is one of the biggest risk factors for developing RLS. It makes sense, then, that as pregnancy progresses and over the course of multiple pregnancies, iron reserves get depleted and RLS ensues. Thankfully, both oral iron and iron infusions (Chapter 5) are considered safe during pregnancy, and there are no significant differences in treatment during pregnancy. Identifying and treating iron deficiency while pregnant can also help prevent your child from developing their own RLS. If the developing fetus does not get enough iron, they might be born with a predisposition to developing RLS as a child.

Another theory is that gestational RLS is related to a deficiency of **folate** (sold in stores as **folic acid**). How folate influences RLS is not clear. Research from the early 2000s found that low folate levels were even more predictive of RLS during pregnancy than low iron. More recent research showed that those with RLS were more likely to have low folate than those without RLS. Still, it's not known if treating the low folate would alleviate the RLS. Nevertheless, since low folate is dangerous for pregnancies in other ways, you should talk to your provider about making sure you get enough folate, which usually involves taking supplements, such as **prenatal vitamins.**

Pregnancy is a time of significant hormone changes, so it is possible that these changes factor into the development of RLS. The hormones **prolactin, estrogen,** and **progesterone** have all been considered possible explanations as to why RLS is so common in pregnancy as they rise throughout the course of pregnancy alongside the rise in RLS symptoms. Thyroid hormone also goes up during pregnancy and has been considered another possible cause. Once pregnancy is over, these hormones decrease along with the severity of RLS.

There are a few problems with the hormonal explanation, though. First, how any of the hormones would cause RLS is not clear. Second, the rise in these hormones occurs in all pregnancies, yet only one quarter of pregnancies are complicated by RLS. There must be other factors. If hormones do play a role, they are interacting with another problem, such as a genetic predisposition or low iron to generate the RLS.

RLS is not the only condition that increases during the third trimester. Other problems, such as heartburn, stuffy nose, and insomnia, are common as well. You may turn to antihistamines to ease the nasal congestion or difficulty sleeping because they are generally considered safe in pregnancy, and they are readily available over the counter. Unfortunately, that can backfire. If you have RLS, antihistamines can trigger it (Chapter 2). If the reason you're not sleeping well is related to RLS, taking an antihistamine may not help you sleep better, as Lisa from the case study at the beginning of this chapter found out.

When Lisa's obstetrician received her email that the diphenhydramine made her sleep worse and learned that her difficulty sleeping was related to uncomfortable legs, she was able to correctly diagnose RLS. She asked Lisa to come by the office to get her iron levels checked. Lisa's levels came back low, so the obstetrician recommended Lisa start daily oral iron supplements, ferrous sulfate 325 mg with vitamin C.

Medications for RLS during pregnancy

Just as it does when you're not pregnant, treating RLS during pregnancy starts with iron (Chapter 5). All of the nonpharmacological therapies also remain available (Chapter 6). After that, though, things get more complicated. Medications you take during pregnancy can, in theory, affect **embryonic** or **fetal** development. Any time you're considering taking a drug while pregnant, including common ones such as caffeine and acetaminophen, you have to weigh the risks with the benefits. The good news is that the common RLS medications are most likely safe enough to take during pregnancy. If your RLS is severe, the benefit of easing your suffering probably outweighs the risks of the medications. This is a conversation that is very important to have with your obstetrician and the provider treating your RLS.

Of the top three classes of medication for RLS—gabapentinoids, dopamine agonists, and opioids (Chapters 7 to 9)—none of them are without some risk.

Gabapentin has many uses in addition to RLS, so more people take it while pregnant than the other common RLS medications. As a result, a lot is known about the effects of gabapentin during pregnancy. With this experience comes confidence that gabapentin is a lower-risk option. Research has shown that **in utero** exposure to gabapentin does not increase the risk of developmental problems. More is known about gabapentin's safety than pregabalin's, so your provider might recommend gabapentin over pregabalin, though pregabalin is likely to have a similar risk profile. The potential side effects of gabapentinoids are the same during pregnancy as they would be if you're not pregnant.

Dopamine agonists are sometimes used during pregnancy, even though less is known about their safety. What is known, though, is mostly reassuring. If you can't take or tolerate gabapentin for any reason, you can talk to your provider about trying dopamine agonists.

Dopamine agonists become a better option later in pregnancy when there is less risk of causing a malformation. Augmentation, the worsening of RLS due to medication, remains a major concern with dopamine agonists and can occur even in the relatively short timeframe of pregnancy.

There are reports of harm from opioids taken earlier in pregnancy, so these drugs are not recommended for use until later, typically during the third trimester. Your goal should be to use them as sparingly as possible. The concern during the third trimester is that if you take opioids regularly, your baby could be born with an opioid dependence, which is a serious though treatable concern.

There are many other possible RLS medications (Chapter 11). Each of these carries its own set of risks. You should definitely avoid certain ones, such as valproic acid and topiramate, during pregnancy. Lamotrigine, on the other hand, is considered about as safe a medication as there is during pregnancy. It is the medication of choice for people with seizures who become pregnant. Clonidine and dipyridamole are not thought to be particularly dangerous during pregnancy, but they do impact blood pressure and bleeding. Your provider might encourage you to stop them if you are feeling lightheaded (clonidine) or approaching your due date (dipyridamole) to reduce your bleeding risk during delivery.

Please remember: these drugs have not been studied for RLS during pregnancy. They've barely been studied for RLS in people who are not pregnant. There is no way to predict if these medications would be of much help to you. For this reason, your provider might want to stick to the classics (gabapentinoids, dopamine agonists, and opioids), because there is much more experience with these.

When weighing the risks and benefits of taking RLS medication during pregnancy, it's important to keep in mind that pregnancy is never risk free. All pregnancies carry the risk of developmental problems or miscarriage. If you choose to take a medication for your RLS and something unexpected or unwanted happens during your pregnancy, you will never know if that would have happened anyway, even if you hadn't taken that medication.

Pregnancy complications, such as miscarriage, are extremely emotionally challenging, and second guessing your decision to take a medication does not help. If you choose to medicate your RLS, you are making the best decision you can with the information you have. An outcome you didn't wish for is not evidence that you made the wrong decision.

Lisa is getting progressively more frustrated with her lack of sleep. She's very concerned about how sleep deprived she will be by the time she delivers. She worries she won't have the energy to care for a newborn if she doesn't sleep more while pregnant. She estimates she's down to just 4 hours of sleep per night despite the iron therapy. Talking it over with her obstetrician, she decides the best course of action is to try gabapentin. Her doctor cautions her that this could lead to drowsiness, but this might be a desirable side effect as it could help her fall asleep better while improving her RLS. Lisa proceeds to take the gabapentin and gets some much-needed sleep.

RLS after pregnancy

If you never had RLS before you became pregnant, good news! Chances are, your RLS will subside rapidly after you deliver. The average time for RLS to resolve after giving birth is about 2 to 4 weeks. The bad news is that you remain at higher risk for developing RLS in the future than if you had never had gestational RLS in the first place. This makes sense if we think of pregnancy as iron-depleting and you never get your brain iron levels back up to where they were before pregnancy. Still, estimates are that about 75% of people who suffer gestational RLS do not go on to a life of RLS.

If you did have RLS prior to pregnancy, that's not likely to change afterward. It might be the same as it was before or it might be worse, but it's not likely to go away unless something else fundamentally changed (maybe you got an iron infusion while pregnant). On the plus side, no longer being pregnant means you have access to a wider selection of treatment options.

Breastfeeding

If you are not breastfeeding, you can resume any medication you might have stopped taking when you became pregnant. If you are breastfeeding, it's important to know what impact any medication you're taking might have on your baby. Thankfully, you can take gabapentinoids and all the seizure drugs in Chapter 11 while breastfeeding. Some medication will likely get to the baby, but there is no evidence that such a low amount would cause your baby any harm. Very little is known about dopamine agonists while breastfeeding. In theory, based on how they work, there is a chance that they could reduce your milk production, but research has not quantified this or revealed what impact, if any, the medication would have on your baby.

Opioids and benzodiazepines present more of a challenge as they readily transfer to breastmilk. As your baby grows, transitions to solid food, and consumes less breastmilk, the risk of harm goes down. But when the baby is small and entirely dependent on breastmilk, they could get a significant dose of medication. This exposure could leave you with an excessively sleepy baby. The doses of these medications for RLS are so low that this is an unlikely outcome, though. It's more likely that you could safely use a low dose of an opioid or benzodiazepine while breastfeeding if this was necessary to control your symptoms.

> Lisa's child is born 3 days before her due date. The child is healthy. A week after returning home from the hospital, Lisa is so busy with the newborn and her other children that she forgets to take her gabapentin before bed. Aside from waking up to feed the baby, she has a good night of sleep. She realizes in the morning that she didn't take the gabapentin and didn't miss it. Her RLS was still mildly present the night before, but she decides that she's done taking the medication and will wait for the rest of the RLS to resolve on its own. She emails her obstetrician to let her know that she is planning to stop gabapentin, and her doctor affirms her decision.

Conclusions

RLS is treatable, even during pregnancy and while breastfeeding. Just like anyone else with RLS, you do not need to suffer. While there are special considerations when it comes to medications, you can work with your provider to get relief. Pregnancy might disrupt your sleep for plenty of other reasons, but your RLS doesn't have to be one of them. And congratulations on the new baby!

CHAPTER 13

RLS with Other Illnesses

In this chapter, you will learn:

- How RLS is managed in hospitalized patients
- How RLS is managed in people with dementia
- How RLS impacts other sleep disorders
- What the relationship is between RLS and ADHD
- What the relationship is between RLS and obesity
- How RLS is managed in people with allergies and immune disorders
- What effect COVID-19 has had on people with RLS

Introduction

While RLS might occur in isolation, most people have RLS and at least one other medical condition. In many instances, these conditions interact to make addressing the RLS even more challenging. This chapter will review RLS in the context of other health conditions you might be dealing with now or in the future. This will include discussions of what it's like to be hospitalized with RLS, how patients with dementia can manage their RLS, and the relationship between RLS and other sleep disorders. The chapter will also cover what is known about the interplay between RLS and attention deficit hyperactivity disorder (ADHD), obesity, and the immune system.

RLS in hospitalized patients

As awful as RLS might make you feel, it is not a condition that will land you in the hospital. You might, however, find yourself hospitalized for any number of other reasons. And if you've ever been in the hospital, you know that there can be some long days and nights in bed. Being stuck in bed is not what people with RLS do best. As if needing to be in the hospital wasn't bad enough, adding RLS to the mix can make it a truly miserable experience.

If you have RLS and need to be hospitalized, there are a variety of issues to be aware of. First, it's possible that your RLS will get worse, not only because you might be immobilized, but also because you're sick. RLS tends to worsen when you get sick, particularly with illnesses that increase inflammation in the body (which is many of them). So now you get the double whammy of your mobility being restricted and your RLS worsening. This will improve once you recover from whatever illness led you to be hospitalized.

The next concern is that you could be exposed to new medications. Antihistamines and antinausea medications are both common triggers for RLS and commonly used in hospitals. The antihistamines fexofenadine and loratadine and the antinausea agent ondansetron can be used instead. These should not exacerbate your RLS. You can ask your hospital medical team if one of these might be an option for you instead of diphenhydramine or promethazine (Chapter 2). If you're having trouble sleeping, your medical team might prescribe an antihistamine to help you sleep. Make sure they know about your RLS so that they can find an alternative that will not worsen your restlessness.

Most of the time, you can continue to take your RLS medication while you're in the hospital. Gabapentin, pregabalin, pramipexole, ropinirole, benzodiazepines, and most opioid medications are readily available in hospital pharmacies. Sometimes, these medications are overlooked when the provider admitting you to the hospital is writing orders for you. If that happens, a gentle reminder about your RLS medication should do the trick.

Methadone and buprenorphine pose unique challenges. Your assigned medical team may have never prescribed these drugs and, frankly, may be nervous to do so. Your medical team needs to be familiar and comfortable with the drugs they are prescribing, though, so they might switch you to an opioid they know better. If you are taking methadone or buprenorphine, this temporary switch will be fine. You will not go into withdrawal if you switch between opioids, although you might notice that other opioids don't treat your RLS as effectively. Keep your medical team apprised of your symptoms so they can adjust your medications if needed.

> Fernando is a 45-year-old man with severe RLS. He takes 5 mg of methadone after dinner each night to control his symptoms, and this works very well for him. He's been on this medication at this dose for 6 years. At his 10-year-old daughter's ice skating birthday party, he slips on the ice and breaks two bones in his lower leg. He's told in the emergency room that he's going to need surgery, and they admit him to the hospital. To treat his pain, the emergency room doctor gives him an injection of hydromorphone, an opioid. Later that night, he meets the surgeon who will operate on his leg the following day. The surgeon asks Fernando why he is on methadone. She has never heard of methadone for RLS and tells him that he can use hydromorphone while he is in the hospital because she is not comfortable prescribing methadone. Fernando is very nervous that he will suffer terrible restlessness without the methadone.

It gets more challenging if you're not allowed to swallow pills or get medication through a feeding tube. All routine RLS medications, aside from rotigotine patches, are given by mouth, so if you cannot take oral medications, you'll need to get your medication another way. None of the gabapentinoids or dopamine agonists come in a patch or an intravenous form, so they're basically off the table as options. Rotigotine patches could be an option, but it's not a medication all hospitals keep on hand. Buprenorphine has a dissolvable form that you might be able to use, but this too might be hard to find in hospital pharmacies.

Injectable options for treating your RLS in the hospital are opioids and benzos. You might already be receiving opioids if you're hospitalized for a condition that causes pain (e.g., surgery). Not all opioids are equally effective in treating RLS, though (Chapter 9). If you are receiving an opioid that is not helping your RLS, you should let your medical team know. There's often no particular reason other than habit that they picked one opioid over another for your pain, and they might be willing to swap the one that isn't helping for one that could help more. Another option if you can't swallow is to use sequential compression devices (Chapter 6). These are common in hospitals because they help prevent the formation of blood clots in the legs. The squeezing of these devices can provide you some much-needed relief.

Being in the hospital is never fun, but RLS doesn't have to magnify your suffering. It is treatable even in the hospital. Since RLS would not be the reason you were admitted to the hospital, your medical team might overlook your RLS as a condition they need to treat while you're there. It is worth advocating for yourself! If your legs are uncomfortable, ask the medical team what can be done about it. Don't assume they know about your RLS or how badly you're suffering. It's okay to speak up. It's GOOD to speak up.

Special considerations for people with RLS and dementia

Dementia and RLS are both very common in older adults. RLS may predispose people to develop dementia (possibly through years of poor sleep), and some causes of dementia can predispose people to RLS (due to reductions in dopamine production). In patients with dementia, it's particularly important to monitor for changes in memory and thinking due to the medications used to treat RLS. Gabapentinoids (Chapter 8) and opioids (Chapter 9) can both cause **cognitive** problems, but benzodiazepines (Chapter 10) are probably the class of drugs that it is most important to avoid.

Giving benzodiazepines to people with dementia can cause particularly severe, even dangerous confusion. Iron replacement (Chapter 5) remains the safest strategy for treatment. If iron levels are sufficient, a dopamine agonist (Chapter 7) at low doses is the next least likely to affect brain functions. These can cause trouble sleeping for some older adults, though. Finally, gabapentinoids and opioids are options, if needed, but careful monitoring of side effects is necessary.

Gail is an 82-year-old woman whose RLS has been treated effectively with 1 mg of clonazepam for 10 years. Her daughter, Pam, has started noticing some changes in Gail's memory. Gail has been forgetting where her keys are. She asks her daughter the same questions throughout the day but doesn't remember the answers. Last week, Gail got disoriented on the way home from her local supermarket and spent 45 minutes driving around her neighborhood before finding her way home. Pam asks Gail if she can accompany her to her next primary care visit, and Gail agrees. Pam tells Gail's primary care provider that she is concerned about Gail's memory and asks about her ongoing use of clonazepam, which she read online can cause dementia. Gail's primary care provider agrees that the symptoms are concerning and that they should work together to find an alternative to clonazepam.

People with RLS tend to be up and moving to address their restlessness. For older adults with dementia, walking around at night, particularly in low light, can lead to falls. Falls are especially dangerous for older adults with dementia and can lead to a cascade of health problems, including death. If you or a loved one have RLS and dementia, treating the RLS to prevent nocturnal walking could help you avoid this outcome.

Diagnosing RLS in people with advanced dementia can be more difficult if the dementia has affected speech abilities. RLS might be causing distress and agitation, but the person suffering from it might not be able to express that verbally. Caregivers might notice repetitive behaviors, such as rubbing the legs or general restlessness. These might be the only clues. While sleep studies are not usually performed for diagnosing RLS, a sleep study that shows frequent leg movements in a patient who otherwise cannot communicate can be used as a surrogate for diagnosing RLS. At the very least, there is no harm in treating low iron levels in patients with dementia who develop overnight agitation to see if the agitation is, in fact, a manifestation of RLS.

RLS in the context of other sleep disorders

RLS, insomnia, and obstructive sleep apnea (OSA) are all very common conditions, so just by coincidence, there are many people who have two or all three of these. RLS also overlaps with some of the less common sleep disorders. There is a possible association between RLS and sleepwalking (Chapter 4). One study even showed a higher rate of RLS in patients with **narcolepsy** than in the general population. This section will focus on RLS and insomnia and RLS and OSA in particular because the link to sleepwalking is not definite and there is very little known about the relationship between narcolepsy and RLS.

Jerry is a 66-year-old man with trouble sleeping. He makes an appointment for himself with a local sleep physician. At the

(Continued)

(Continued)

appointment, Jerry tells the physician that he has been having trouble falling and staying asleep. "I toss and turn and never seem to get comfortable," he says. "Eventually I fall asleep, but then, I wake up to use the bathroom and when I get back into bed, I toss and turn all over again, so it takes me an hour or two to fall back asleep. I get so little sleep that I'm exhausted all the time!" The sleep doctor asks about Jerry's sleep schedule and bedtime habits as well as about symptoms of RLS. He also asks Jerry if he snores. Jerry provides positive responses to both the RLS screening questions and to the snoring. The doctor then explains to Jerry that there are probably multiple sleep disorders at work, and they need to address each of them before Jerry will be able to sleep well.

RLS and insomnia

It can be challenging to differentiate trouble sleeping from RLS and trouble sleeping from insomnia. Insomnia is defined as difficulty falling asleep, difficulty staying asleep, or waking up earlier than desired despite having the opportunity and environment to sleep. If you have insomnia and struggle to fall asleep, it gives your legs a chance to start getting restless. Alternatively, if you get into bed and your restless legs keep you from falling asleep, it can feel like insomnia. Some people with insomnia toss and turn and generally feel uncomfortable, but that isn't necessarily RLS. Sorting all of this out with your provider will help them determine the best treatment plan.

Many people with RLS will have symptoms while relaxing in the evening before bed. If this sensation transfers to the bedroom and persists to the point of preventing sleep, it's clear that the RLS needs to be treated to facilitate sleep. If the treatment helps your legs but not your sleep, though, you might have insomnia also. This is an important distinction. Judging the success of your RLS treatment by how quickly you fall asleep at night might make you think the RLS medication isn't working. RLS treatments are just supposed to calm your legs down, though, not put you to sleep. Remember this when you are reporting to your provider on how well your treatment is working. You don't want to stop an effective RLS medication because you were expecting too much from it.

If you have insomnia independent of your RLS, it must be treated as its own problem. Insomnia is best treated through a process called cognitive behavioral therapy for insomnia (CBT-I). One great thing about CBT-I is that you can sleep better without the need to take more pills. In fact, sleep medicine providers usually do everything possible to avoid prescribing sleeping pills. CBT-I can help you identify and change thoughts and behaviors that impair your sleep.

While some people report lifelong sleep problems, for many people with insomnia, there was a trigger that created the sleep problems. This trigger could be RLS. Have you grown so accustomed to struggling to fall asleep when you get into bed that you expect it to happen? If so, you might be enacting a self-fulfilling prophecy. People who expect to sleep poorly usually do. When night after night you get into bed and feel uncomfortable due to your legs, you start to associate the bed as a location where you feel uncomfortable. Then, even if your RLS improves, your brain still associates the bed with discomfort, and you don't fall asleep. This is called **classical conditioning** (Figure 13.1). One of the goals of CBT-I is to help you break this conditioning and restore the bed as a place of comfort and relaxation. This only works once the RLS is under control, though. It's usually more effective to treat the RLS first so that your insomnia treatment is not limited by your RLS.

RLS and obstructive sleep apnea

The trouble with RLS for patients with OSA is that it can interfere with treatment. OSA causes your airway to partially or fully close during sleep, temporarily preventing breathing. It is most commonly treated

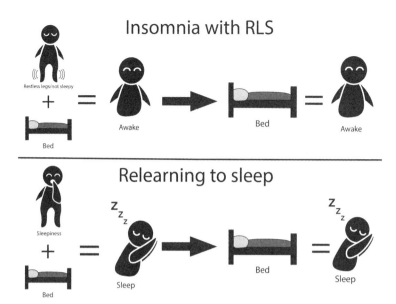

FIGURE 13.1 The person on the top has RLS and gets into bed when feeling restless, leading to being awake in bed. This conditions the person to be awake in bed even if the RLS disappears. The person on the bottom has treated their RLS. This person gets into bed when sleepy and falls asleep. This helps pair the bed with sleep so that the bed becomes a trigger for sleep instead of for being awake. (Figure credit: Adaora Spector)

with a continuous positive airway pressure (CPAP) machine. Using a CPAP machine requires a person to wear a mask that is attached by a hose to a machine that sits by the bed. Patients with RLS can struggle to lie in bed with a CPAP machine on because they have to get up and down too often, and taking the mask on and off can be troublesome.

Treating OSA is critically important, though. Not only is untreated OSA associated with many long-term health problems, but also one study showed that treatment of OSA resulted in improved RLS symptoms in 74% of study subjects. Win-win! You can be healthier and have improved RLS from using a CPAP machine. Even better, CPAP machines just provide pressurized air, so this is possibly the safest means of treating RLS there is (no drugs!). CPAP isn't an option if you have RLS without OSA, but if you do, using your CPAP machine regularly is a great strategy.

Of the medications used for RLS, opioids pose the most potential risk to someone with OSA. Taking a medication that can suppress breathing when you already have trouble breathing in your sleep can be a dangerous combination. Additionally, taking opioids can lead to central sleep apnea (Chapter 9), which can complicate your treatment for OSA. Your sleep apnea care provider can monitor your breathing by looking at the data from your CPAP machine to see if this is happening and suggest treatment strategies if it is.

RLS in the context of ADHD

ADHD and RLS not only co-occur but also might share some of the same changes in the brain. Research has found that 12% to 44% of people with ADHD have RLS and 11% to 26% of people with RLS have ADHD. This is too high of an overlap to just be a coincidence. Since both conditions tend to run strongly in families, there is a possibility that they either share the same genetic cause or are caused by different genes that happen to co-occur in the same families.

The prominent ADHD symptom of **inattention** is also a symptom of sleep deprivation. It is possible that some people diagnosed with ADHD are actually suffering from poor sleep. In this case, treating the RLS and improving sleep quality might reduce or eliminate the symptoms that led to the diagnosis of ADHD. Others who have both ADHD and RLS might notice improved symptom control of the ADHD by getting better sleep.

ADHD, like RLS, is frequently treated with medications that increase activity in the dopamine pathways (Chapter 3). Low functioning in this pathway could be a shared mechanism for both conditions. Dopamine neurons are present in many places in the brain, so it could be that the specific location in the brain where the dopamine dysfunction is most prominent determines which symptoms you have. Norepinephrine has also been associated with both RLS and ADHD. In fact, clonidine, a medication that reduces norepinephrine, can treat both RLS and ADHD (Chapter 11).

For people with severe ADHD, it can be difficult to fall asleep. This is often described by patients as having a hyperactive mind in bed. This might even co-occur with the hyperactive legs of people with RLS. Low doses of ADHD medications, which typically take the form of **stimulants** such as methylphenidate or amphetamines, can paradoxically relax people with ADHD and help them fall asleep. No research has examined these ADHD medications for the treatment of RLS, and it's very unlikely that your provider would offer you a stimulant to calm your legs at night, but the overlap is intriguing and could be an inspiration for future research.

Aside from the overlap with dopamine, there's a possible link between ADHD and RLS when it comes to iron. One small study showed that children with ADHD symptoms improved with iron supplements, again supporting the idea that there are similar brain processes involved in both conditions. Other research, though, has not found a link between iron levels and ADHD, so the role of iron in this condition is not as well established as it is for RLS. For now, we know that treating your RLS with iron therapy will not hurt your ADHD, and it might help.

Brandon is a 42-year-old man who has been treated for ADHD since middle school. His primary care provider referred him to a neurologist to evaluate for possible RLS after Brandon described uncomfortable feelings in his legs at night that make him want to kick them. The neurologist agrees that this is likely RLS. Brandon chuckles when he receives the diagnosis of RLS, telling the neurologist that he's just like his father, who also has ADHD and RLS.

RLS in the context of obesity

There has been a steady increase in the rate of **obesity** across the world over the past 60 years. Obesity increases your risk of RLS, so it's possible the **prevalence** of RLS has also increased over the same period, but it has not been tracked. One possible reason for the obesity-RLS association is that obesity causes increased inflammation in the body, and inflammation can worsen RLS. It's also possible that both conditions are caused by alterations in dopamine pathways. A good deal of research has established that obesity can result from abnormal dopamine-related control of appetite and eating. Thus, obesity and RLS could share a cause.

Jacqueline is a 55-year-old woman who was referred to a sleep medicine clinic to address her RLS. She was diagnosed with RLS about 20 years ago, but it was mild, and she was able to avoid taking medications. Now it has gotten to the point that she would like to consider starting treatment. The nurse practitioner in the sleep clinic reviews her history with her and discovers that 5 years ago, Jacqueline underwent surgery to help her lose weight. The nurse practitioner suggests that they start by checking iron because of the association between low iron and RLS. Jacqueline tells the nurse practitioner that she has been taking iron supplements by mouth ever since her surgery. The nurse practitioner instructs Jacqueline not to take her iron supplement for a day and then have her iron levels checked in the morning before breakfast. The labs come back indicating that Jacqueline is iron deficient, and the nurse practitioner recommends an iron infusion.

Further evidence that obesity has a role to play in the cause of RLS is that weight loss can improve RLS. In a small study of 14 patients undergoing surgery for weight loss, 12 of them were able to stop medications for RLS within 12 months. Weight loss surgery comes with potential complications, though, such as a reduced ability to absorb iron and a tendency to become iron deficient. If you have had weight loss surgery and continue to have RLS in the setting of iron deficiency, you would be a good candidate for an iron infusion rather than oral iron supplements.

If you have both RLS and obesity, there are side effects from two common classes of medication to look out for. First, gabapentinoids are associated with weight gain. Even if you don't gain weight, they could make it harder to lose weight if that is your goal. Thankfully, research suggests that this is not a common side effect. Of the two, pregabalin probably causes more weight gain than gabapentin, but there is no way to predict which one might cause more weight gain for you. If you are among the people who gain weight from gabapentinoids, the weight gain can be significant, which is why you need careful monitoring so that you can stop the drug before the weight gain is substantial.

The second class of medication that causes trouble is dopamine agonists. These drugs cause eating-related impulse control disorders (Chapter 7). Even though dopamine agonists don't cause weight gain directly, they will if they take away your ability to regulate your food intake. Like all the impulse control disorders, it's critical to let your provider know right away if this develops so that you can be weaned off the medication quickly and safely.

RLS in the context of allergies and immune system disorders

If you have allergies—to medications, foods, pollen, or all of the above—you're probably familiar with antihistamines. They can be lifesaving, both figuratively and literally. Unfortunately, many antihistamines cause problems for people with RLS. Stick to the specific set of antihistamines that do not affect the brain and thus do not worsen RLS (Chapter 2). Your best bet is to use fexofenadine or loratadine. On the box, look for "nondrowsy," as that's your sign that it doesn't affect the brain.

Although not the same as a drug allergy, other conditions that cause medication intolerances, such as **mast cell activation syndrome (MCAS)** or **multiple chemical sensitivity**, can also impact RLS therapy. If you have one of these conditions, you might struggle to tolerate any medications at all. If you have MCAS, it is important to avoid medications that trigger your reactions. Of the RLS medications, opioids are most likely to do this, and of the opioids, morphine and oxycodone are the ones you should most avoid. Gabapentinoids tend to be better tolerated and would be considered first-line therapy after iron supplementation. In the case of multiple chemical sensitivity, it is not possible to predict which medications will be better tolerated than others. Unfortunately, this means trial and error to sort out what the best drug is for you or maximizing the nonpharmacological treatments to avoid taking any additional medications (Chapter 6).

RLS and COVID-19

Even several years after the onset of the **COVID-19 pandemic**, research on the disease is still in its infancy, but it did not take long to recognize that the pandemic exacerbated RLS. Many people were no longer leaving their houses or getting regular exercise. Jobs that used to require moving around an office were converted to day-long video conferencing at a desk. Being sedentary is bad for RLS, and the pandemic made it harder to avoid a sedentary lifestyle.

Beyond lifestyle changes, for those who caught the virus, it might have played a role in causing or exacerbating RLS. There are reports of new-onset RLS in the setting of COVID-19 illness as well as a higher rate of RLS in people with persistent symptoms after COVID-19, commonly referred to as "**long COVID**." In one study, the rate of

RLS nearly tripled from before getting sick to having long COVID. And while the COVID-19 vaccines are by far the best way to avoid life-threatening COVID-19 illness, there are reports that a small percentage of people developed RLS after vaccination.

When both the virus and the vaccines (which do not contain the virus) can cause the same symptom, it's likely that the immune system is the common denominator. While it's not known what aspects of the body's immune response can cause or worsen RLS, it is clear that inflammation can worsen RLS. It will take another few years to determine if COVID-associated RLS is temporary or persistent. Most likely, the RLS will resolve over time, as this is what happens in other illnesses, and neither viral nor vaccine-related RLS will become a lifelong problem.

Conclusions

RLS does not occur in a vacuum. Many people with RLS have at least one other health issue going on. Regardless of what those problems might be, your RLS can be managed. You should never be told that there's nothing to be done about your RLS because of any other medical condition. You always deserve to have your RLS addressed and under control.

CHAPTER 14

Periodic Limb Movements

In this chapter, you will learn:

- What are periodic limb movements
- What is the association between periodic limb movements and RLS
- When do periodic limb movements become a problem
- What can be done to reduce periodic limb movements

Introduction

Periodic limb movements of sleep (PLMS) and RLS are different entities (Chapter 1). This book is about RLS, not PLMS, but there is a very large overlap. Up to 90% of people with RLS will have PLMS, while 30% of people with PLMS will have RLS. RLS gets more attention from researchers, has more name recognition among the public, and makes the people who live with it markedly more miserable than people living with PLMS who do not have RLS. Nevertheless, PLMS are important in their own right, and it's unlikely anyone is going to write a whole book about them, so this chapter will provide a deeper look at this phenomenon. We will explore when PLMS might be considered a problem and what can be done about them if they start to interfere with sleep.

"Periodic limb movements" is a fancy term for a type of leg jerk. A leg jerk during sleep is considered significant if it is brief (0.5 to

10 seconds long), is at least moderately forceful (based on electrical monitoring), and does not occur immediately following a breathing problem. If the reason your legs are jerking is because you can't breathe, that doesn't count. The leg jerks can occur in one or both legs. These movements often occur in a series with a generally consistent amount of time between the events. In other words, the time period between events is about the same, leading to the name "periodic" limb movements. Don't confuse this with the colloquial definition of periodic, which would imply "occasional." The period between leg movements ranges from every 5 seconds to every 90 seconds. Bedpartners can often accurately report their partner's rhythm, as they lie awake counting the seconds between jerks.

Jerome is a 79-year-old man who is seeing a physician assistant in the sleep clinic for his first follow-up visit after starting treatment for obstructive sleep apnea. He is very pleased to report that he's doing great. He is waking up fewer times per night to use the bathroom and his daytime energy is back to where it was 20 years earlier. He hasn't felt this good in years, he says. He has one remaining question for the physician assistant, though. "I was looking at the report of my sleep study, and it says that my PLMS were 32 per hour. What are PLMS and what do I need to do about them?" The physician assistant explains to Jerome what "PLMS" means and reassures him that since he is feeling so good, there is nothing he needs to do about this finding.

PLMS are very common. By age 65, it is estimated that 40% of the population has them. PLMS are not a disease, and for most people, they are probably meaningless. If they don't bother you, ignore them. That might be easier said than done for your bedpartner, but from the perspective of the person doing the jerking, treatment is discouraged. One day we might discover that PLMS are more dangerous than we think they are, but for now, unless you have symptoms, leave them alone.

PLMS versus PLMD

If you do have symptoms related to your PLMS, which could include frequent nighttime awakenings, nonrestorative or unrestful sleep, or daytime sleepiness, you could qualify for a diagnosis of periodic limb movement disorder (PLMD). For this diagnosis, you would have at least 15 PLMS per hour plus some sort of impairment in functioning as a result. Some people have well over 100 per hour. Since so many people have PLMS that cause no problems, it can be very difficult to determine when your leg jerks are responsible for your symptoms. Generally, your providers will address all other sleep problems first, particularly sleep apnea. Then, if you are still struggling with sleep and sleepiness, it is reasonable to target your legs.

> Amara is a 35-year-old woman who went to her primary care doctor to discuss her snoring and daytime sleepiness. She tells her primary care provider that her bedpartner is concerned that she has sleep apnea because of how loudly she snores. The primary care provider refers her to the sleep lab for a sleep study, and Amara sees a sleep doctor to get her results the following week. The sleep doctor tells her that although she snored a lot, the test was negative for sleep apnea. He also tells her that she had 72 PLMS per hour, of which 20 per hour disrupted her sleep. He suggests that since the test showed no sleep apnea but she felt so sleepy during the day, they should try treating her legs to get them to quiet down overnight.

When a leg jerk arouses you from sleep, it's called a **limb movement arousal**. These arousals are often so brief that you can't remember them, so there's no way to judge for yourself how frequently this is happening. If you do a sleep study in a sleep lab, you'll get a score for your periodic limb movement frequency as well as your limb movement arousal frequency. It's common to have far more limb movements than limb movement arousals because most limb movements do not disturb your sleep. (Your bedpartner's sleep, on the other hand, is a different story). For the diagnosis of PLMD, it's the periodic limb movement frequency that counts, not the frequency of arousals. This may seem counterintuitive because it would make sense that the degree of sleep disruption would matter more than the frequency of leg jerks, but that's not the way it's done. It will not surprise me if that changes one day.

PLMS are defined by the actions of the legs, but your arms can jerk too. One reason that PLMS are defined as leg movements and not arm movements is because only the legs are routinely monitored during sleep studies. It's hard to know how often the arms are affected if they're not even recorded. Even though the name of the condition is "limb" movements, leg movements are what count.

Labeling RLS versus PLMS versus PLMD

The terms RLS, PLMS, and PLMD have official definitions, but they are sometimes used more casually in provider office visit notes. Let's disentangle these terms so you have a clear understanding of what's what.

Officially, if you have RLS and PLMS, only the RLS is diagnosed because the PLMS are considered a component of the RLS. You don't need two diagnoses. Likewise, you can't officially have RLS and PLMD for the same reason. PLMS that cause no harm are more of an interesting observation than a diagnosis because, by definition, they aren't leading to any major consequences. PLMD is only diagnosed when you have symptoms from your PLMS but you don't have RLS.

Providers who use these terms more casually might write diagnoses such as "RLS/PLMS" or "RLS/PLMD" as a way of noting that you have both issues even though, technically, RLS is the formal diagnosis. The lingo may be confusing, but if you see these terms in your medical record, you will now know what they mean.

Treating PLMD

Medications for PLMD are the same as the medications for RLS. In fact, the guidelines for treatment put forward by organizations such as the American Academy of Sleep Medicine include both RLS and PLMD in the same document. Little research has been done on how best to treat PLMD or what the response to treatment is. For example, it's not known whether reducing PLMS improves the symptoms of PLMD. It seems logical that it would, but that research has never actually been done.

The primary source of information we have about treating PLMD comes from the studies of RLS in which researchers looked at reductions in PLMS in addition to improvement in RLS symptoms. Of the RLS medications, the dopamine agonists (Chapter 7) seem to reduce PLMS the most. Gabapentinoids and opioids (Chapters 8 and 9) are also effective, but not quite as effective as the dopamine agonists. One easy decision, though, is to start iron therapy (Chapter 5) if your levels are low.

Amara gets her iron levels checked and they are low. Her sleep doctor recommends iron therapy before starting prescription medication. Amara starts ferrous sulfate 325 mg daily. She has trouble tolerating this due to constipation, so she and her sleep doctor decide that she should get an iron infusion. Two months later, she returns to the sleep clinic to report that she is feeling much better.

If you and your provider opt to start medication for PLMD, it's not clear that you will feel any better even if your PLMS entirely resolve. This is because you can't know in advance of treatment if your symptoms are due to PLMD or not. And there are only a few ways to know if your PLMS are being treated: your bedpartner tells you so, you have another sleep study, or your bedcovers are no longer disheveled in the morning.

If you get to the point that you are having a follow-up sleep study and your PLMS are gone, yet you are still sleeping poorly or feeling badly during the day, you and your provider might reconsider the diagnosis of PLMD. At that point, it's likely that something else is affecting your sleep and the PLMS noted on your initial sleep study were not the culprit. Seeing a sleep medicine specialist can help you sort through this.

CHAPTER 15

RLS in Vulnerable Populations

In this chapter, you will learn:

- What constitutes a vulnerable population
- What barriers vulnerable populations face to receiving care for RLS

Introduction

Regardless of the type of health system a country has, there are always some people who have better access to health care than others. Those who are at higher risk of disease or of receiving inadequate medical care are considered **vulnerable**. Sometimes, this is a simple matter of geography. If you're having an emergency and live close to a hospital, you can get to a hospital faster. Your odds of surviving a medical emergency drop as the distance to a major medical center increases. In the United States, patients living in rural areas find themselves in this vulnerable position. But living close to a hospital is no guarantee of rapid care. If there are not enough hospitals in a densely populated area, you might get to the hospital and still not receive timely care due to long wait times. Thus, patients living in urban areas can also be vulnerable.

Children and older adults are also vulnerable populations due to their higher risk of certain diseases as well as their potential for dependence on others. People with disabilities, migrants and refugees, members of racial and ethnic minority groups, low-income groups (including those with and without stable housing), and sexual and gender minorities can all be considered vulnerable in certain contexts. This chapter will address how some of these vulnerable groups are at risk of receiving inadequate care for their RLS.

Rural populations

For patients living in rural areas, access to health care can be a major challenge. Finding a primary care provider is challenging enough. Finding a specialist with expertise in RLS could be downright impossible. Thankfully, there has been a big change in the care of rural patients with the explosion of **telehealth** during the COVID-19 pandemic. Now, patients can be treated without having to leave their homes. You do need a reliable internet connection for this to be successful, so telehealth does not solve the problem entirely. Most people do have access to broadband internet, though, and more are getting it every day. Some rural locations have opened telehealth centers where you can have your telehealth visit if you don't have fast internet access at home.

Frank is an 81-year-old man who owns a convenience store and gas station along a stretch of state highway in a large, western state. Frank stopped driving a year ago because his vision had worsened, and it was no longer safe. Frank has severe RLS. He has been taking pramipexole for the past 4 years, but the maximum dose of 0.5 mg per night is not effective anymore. The nurse practitioner in the local clinic recommended he see a neurologist for more advanced care, but the nearest neurologist is in a clinic in the city where Frank's son works, nearly an hour away. Frank tells the nurse

(Continued)

(Continued)

practitioner that he will only be able to attend this appointment if his son can get the time off from work to drive out to get him and take him home afterward. He's also worried that his store will have to stay closed for most of the day, which will cost him substantial revenue. The nurse practitioner offers a solution. If he can get back to her clinic, she can arrange for him to see the neurologist with the telehealth equipment they have in the office.

Some of the medications prescribed for RLS are controlled substances, which means they are more tightly regulated. The rules for the prescription of controlled substances during telehealth appointments are heavily debated. Some people worry that nefarious online groups will inappropriately prescribe these medications to too many people, increasing the risk of drug abuse and overdose or drug diversion, the reselling of medications to those without a prescription. Many patient advocates, however, argue that restricting the prescription of controlled substances to in-person visits creates a particular hardship for people living in rural areas who might struggle to get to these appointments.

Beyond access to care, rural areas also see higher rates of certain conditions that can exacerbate RLS, such as cigarette smoking, kidney disease, and sedentary lifestyles. Additionally, the more medical conditions your provider must address at your appointment, the less time there is for treating your RLS. If your rural location makes it difficult to access a provider to care for your RLS, you can begin by working with your local provider to improve your overall health. Treatment of some of these other conditions can improve your RLS also. You can also begin your own therapy with any of the strategies that can improve RLS without medications (Chapter 6).

Low-income, urban populations

For people earning lower incomes, living in an urban area comes with its own vulnerabilities. Many health care facilities cluster in higher-income areas. This puts low-income groups in a similar quandary to rural patients: how to get to the office to see a provider in person. Even with access to public transportation, it can take an hour or 2 to get across a congested city. For hourly wage workers, taking this much time off to see a doctor could cause substantial financial hardship from lost wages or even loss of the job. Telehealth can be critical for access to care, even if you only live a few miles from the clinic.

Priya is a 28-year-old woman living in a large city on the East Coast of the United States. She was referred by her primary care provider to a neurologist for treatment of her RLS. Priya tried to get an appointment with the neurologist near the store where she works as a salesclerk, but she wasn't accepting new patients. Priya called the next closest neurologist and learned that he wasn't in her insurance network. She then called her insurance company and got the name of an in-network neurologist. Priya planned out her route to this third neurologist's office. It was across town, which would require two buses and a half-mile walk. It would take her about 90 minutes to get there, so she would have to take half a day off work to go. She asked for the time off, but her boss told her that since she had only been there for 6 weeks, she was not allowed time off. At this point, Priya gave up and never made it to the neurologist.

Priya's story also highlights issues surrounding health insurance. Finding an in-network provider can be a challenge, and that assumes you have insurance at all. Even if you can get seen in the office, there's still the trouble of paying for treatment. Then, if you have prescription drug coverage as part of your insurance, getting your medication covered might require **prior authorization**, a common tactic used by insurance companies to avoid paying for the treatment recommended by your provider. For RLS, the two medications most frequently impacted by the prior authorization process are gabapentin enacarbil and rotigotine patches. Even if your provider is able to get these approved, your **copay** might still make these drugs too expensive.

For those without insurance, there are still ways to get medications. Some drug companies will provide medications to those who qualify based on income. And there are several websites that now offer coupons for medications that do not require insurance. These coupons can be very helpful. In fact, sometimes the coupon price is lower than the price with insurance. Your pharmacist or your provider can help you find these coupons. Over-the-counter medications, such as iron supplements, are not typically covered by insurance, but thankfully the cost of these pills can be as low as 4 cents per day.

Racial and ethnic minority populations

Although White patients are most likely to develop RLS, patients from racial and ethnic minority groups can also suffer from this condition. These groups could face barriers in both diagnosis and treatment. When a condition is substantially more common in one racial group, patients in other groups can be overlooked when they have the same condition. There are examples of this problem throughout health care. **Cystic fibrosis**, a genetic disease that affects predominantly the lungs, for instance, is so much more common in White people that those in another racial group are much older by the time their disease is recognized, with the potential for permanent damage to the body in the meantime. **Sickle cell disease**, a genetic blood disorder, by contrast, is much more common among Black people, so it goes unrecognized in other racial groups. Doctors aren't perfect, and diagnoses get missed.

> Jerry is a 28-year-old man who identifies as African American. He has had a disease of his intestines for the past 12 years that causes him to have bloody bowel movements. Losing blood this way has led to a depletion of his iron on several occasions in the past. At his recent primary care visit, he mentions to his doctor that his legs are bothering him at night. His doctor suggests that he elevate his legs in the evening to reduce any swelling. Jerry tries this over the next week, but it makes his legs feel worse. Jerry's doctor next orders an electromyogram with a nerve test to see if Jerry has neuropathy. When this test comes back normal, he tells Jerry that there doesn't appear to be anything wrong with his legs, but he'll refer Jerry to a neurologist in case there's anything he's missing. The neurologist hears Jerry's story, suspects Jerry has RLS, and orders iron tests. Jerry's ferritin level is 5 µg/L, which the neurologist explains is very low. He suspects that raising Jerry's iron level will improve his legs and orders an iron infusion for Jerry. Within 2 weeks of the infusion, Jerry's legs already feel much better.

Health care providers are taught to see patterns, and when some element, like skin color, doesn't fit a pattern, a diagnosis can get inadvertently overlooked. In Jerry's case, his primary care doctor took Jerry's concerns seriously, attempted to help him, but did not recognize the diagnosis. Jerry was fortunate to have a primary doctor who cared enough to try to help him. It's impossible to know for sure if Jerry's race played a role in the missed diagnosis or not, but these types of occurrences are common enough to suspect it was relevant. If you identify as a member of a group other than White and live in the United States, you might need to encourage your provider to consider a diagnosis of RLS because RLS is so much less common in people of other races.

There could also be barriers in treatment. There is a common misperception that racial and ethnic minority groups, particularly Black Americans, are more likely to use illicit drugs, such as heroin. In fact, White Americans are far more likely to abuse opioids than Black Americans. This bias can result in providers having greater reluctance to prescribe opioids to Black patients. Research has shown that pain is treated with fewer opioids or lower doses in Black patients, so the same might be true for RLS. This could leave Black patients inadequately treated.

Sexual and gender minorities

Patients who identify as gay, lesbian, bisexual, or transgender are more likely than their heterosexual and cisgender counterparts to avoid health care settings due to legitimate concerns about discrimination or harassment. This can lead to underdiagnosis and undertreatment of many conditions, including RLS. In addition, members of sexual or gender minority groups are more likely to misuse or abuse opioids, both prescription and illicit. This could lead providers to shy away from prescribing opioid therapy, even when indicated for severe RLS. If you are a member of a sexual or gender minority group, finding a health care provider in a welcoming clinic is important for your care. Some health care institutions are now publicly identifying providers who either identify as a member of a sexual or gender minority themselves or consider themselves allies to help you find a provider with whom you can feel comfortable.

People with disabilities

There are many different kinds of disabilities. Some are visible, and some aren't. Some are physical, some are cognitive, and some are psychological, to name a few. Physical disabilities, specifically those that limit mobility, can provide a unique barrier when it comes to accessing care. Getting to an appointment might require reliance on certain kinds of transportation that can accommodate a mobility aid, such as a wheelchair. Once at the office, getting into the building if there are stairs and navigating crowded waiting rooms or small spaces can be a significant challenge. Patients with physical disabilities can benefit greatly from the availability of telehealth appointments.

For patients with cognitive disabilities, language difficulties might make communicating the symptoms impossible. Agitation or increased fidgeting at night might be the only clue to a caregiver that something is wrong. It can be extremely challenging to determine that RLS is the cause. This means that people with cognitive disabilities might never make it to an RLS provider at all.

Summary

Vulnerable populations face challenges throughout the health care system, starting with recognition of the need to see a health care provider, followed by accessing a provider, being treated respectfully and appropriately in the health care setting, and obtaining proper therapy. All patients face these hurdles to some degree, but for vulnerable patients, these obstacles can be more difficult or even impossible to overcome.

RLS poses some unique challenges to vulnerable populations. For instance, it's necessary to overcome the bias and stigma in the prescription of opioid medications, which are commonly used for RLS. It can also be difficult for providers to give RLS the time it deserves during a brief clinic visit, so it gets pushed aside to deal with other issues, such as high blood pressure or diabetes, even if RLS is the one that is bothering you the most. For patients with easier access to care, a second visit to focus specifically on the RLS would be easier to come by, but for rural or lower-income patients, one visit per year might be all they can muster.

There is room for cautious optimism with the rise of telehealth, expansion of high-speed internet, proliferation of drug discount programs, efforts to end stigmas against opioid users, and accelerating momentum to reform the prior authorization process. Each of these will improve the care of vulnerable populations. Sadly, even with all of these reforms, the inequities in the health care system will persist as long as we have inequities in society that create a higher burden of disease in these vulnerable groups.

.

CHAPTER 16

Information for Loved Ones and Caregivers

In this chapter, you will learn:

- What loved ones can do to help people with RLS
- How RLS can impact loved ones

Introduction

If you have never experienced RLS and are reading this book because you want to better understand what your loved one with RLS is going through—wow! They are so lucky to have you in their lives. If you are the one with RLS and are reading this chapter to get some ideas as to what to tell your loved one about your RLS, that's great too, but please keep in mind that when I address you, the reader, in this chapter, I am addressing those who have not experienced RLS personally but care about someone who has. If you skipped straight to this chapter to get advice as a caregiver, I would encourage you to read more about RLS in the earlier chapters of this book to have a better understanding of what your loved one is experiencing and why.

Inge and George have been married for 40 years. For the past 10 years, George has been dealing with severe RLS. Inge knows

(Continued)

(Continued)

that George carries this diagnosis, but she does not know what it is. She works full time and has not attended any of George's medical visits where the diagnosis has been discussed. She asked George to explain it to her, but he says that all he knows is that his legs bother him when he tries to sit down in the evening. He does not feel comfortable explaining to Inge why he has this sensation. Inge is frustrated because she sees George suffering and doesn't know what to do about it.

Take it seriously!

Reading this book puts you a step ahead of Inge. By now, you know what RLS is and what causes it (Chapters 1 to 3). It's not George's fault that he has a hard time explaining RLS to Inge. RLS is difficult for many patients to describe. The English language doesn't seem to have a word that captures the unpleasant but not painful sensation people experience. You should not confuse the lack of pain for lack of misery, though. One of the worst things you can do is minimize the amount of distress this causes your loved one. Just because you can't see anything wrong in their legs does not mean they aren't feeling it. This is an invisible disease. Imagine feeling so restless that you can't sit down to watch TV or read in the evening. Imagine dreading going to a movie and being trapped in the middle of a row, unable to get up and move if needed. People adapt their lives around this condition, avoiding long flights or car rides, or any situation that might require prolonged sitting. Please, do not underestimate how bad this can get.

Identifying causes of RLS

One of your jobs as a loved one or caregiver is to help identify potential causes of RLS so they can be reported to their health care provider. If your loved one is consuming alcohol, tobacco, or caffeine, helping them quit can be very beneficial. If you do the shopping, stop buying these items. Encourage your loved one to seek help with alcohol or tobacco addictions for which several medical therapies exist to help maintain abstinence. Without nagging, remind your loved one if they are about to grab a caffeinated beverage in the afternoon without realizing it. Finally, help your loved one remember to report all of the associated chronic illnesses (such as kidney failure, multiple sclerosis, stroke, neuropathy, heart failure, or vitamin D deficiency) to the clinician caring for their RLS so these can be appropriately addressed.

Treating RLS as a team

Although RLS is most frequently treated with iron supplementation or prescription medications, there are actually many nonpharmacological treatments that can help, and this is a great way for a caregiver to provide support. Moderate daily exercise is important to reduce RLS symptoms, so you can both encourage and join your loved one in an exercise routine. One of the best ways to reduce RLS is through massage. If you really want to do them a favor, ask your loved one if you can rub their legs for them. People with RLS often love having someone massage their legs. With the understanding that you can't massage someone all evening, another strategy you can employ is distraction. Play games, do puzzles, or get up and dance. Do something that is not just sitting passively and watching TV. The mental or physical stimulation can help reduce their suffering.

Monitoring medications

Sometimes RLS requires medications to get it under control even after eliminating the triggers and replacing iron. There are many choices, and you can be a big help to your loved one by helping to keep track of how they do on each medication they try. Keep a record. Is it effective? Do they have side effects? What doses have they been on?

Caregivers can be particularly helpful in monitoring side effects of dopamine agonists (Chapter 7). Problem number one is that these drugs can actually cause worsening of RLS over time. The symptoms might start earlier in the day or spread to other body parts. This is called augmentation, and the best way to treat it is to get off the drug that's causing it. Your loved one might not recognize this is happening, but if you notice that they're taking their medication earlier than they used to or they're starting to have symptoms before dinner, you could suggest augmentation as a possibility.

The other major problem is impulse control disorders. You might notice your loved one displaying uncharacteristic behavior. The common types are compulsive eating, compulsive shopping, compulsive gambling, and compulsive pornography consumption or other sexual behaviors. Compulsive means they can't stop even when you and they know they should. This is not their fault, and it's critically important that their provider know this is happening to be able to wean off the medication.

If you don't recognize the association between these medications and these behaviors, they can go on a long time with substantial damage to you and your loved one's lives. Your role as a loved one is to be on the lookout for these changes, which can start at any time after being on this medication. If the medication is stopped, the behaviors usually stop within 1 or 2 months.

Lucy is a 94-year-old woman who lives alone and is generally able to care for herself. She stopped driving 2 months ago due to vision problems, so her daughter accompanies her to her medical appointments now. Lucy is treated for RLS with pramipexole 0.5 mg. At the visit with her RLS provider, she notes that this dose is not helping as much as it used to. The doctor explains that she is reluctant to increase the dose

(Continued)

(Continued)

further because it can cause more trouble down the road. Lucy asks the doctor to reconsider because pramipexole "was like magic" when she first started taking it, as her symptoms went away quickly. The doctor responds that in addition to possibly causing her to have even more symptoms, higher doses are more likely to trigger compulsive behaviors, like gambling or shopping. "Mom!" Lucy's daughter exclaims. "Maybe that's why you've been buying all of those things you don't need from the TV shopping network!"

Gabapentinoids are now the preferred treatment for RLS rather than the dopamine agonists. The risks tend to be lower than for the other classes of medication. If your loved one is experiencing sedation, it's important to keep them safe until the medication effect wears off. This means no driving. You can also help monitor for depression as your loved one might not recognize the change in their own mood as quickly as you do. Encourage your loved one to let their provider know about these side effects.

Opioids, also known as narcotics, are frequently used for severe RLS that has not responded to other treatments. These include drugs such as methadone, buprenorphine, oxycodone, hydrocodone, tramadol, codeine, and morphine. Opioids are scary. There is an opioid crisis that is taking the lives of hundreds of thousands of people. You should not take these drugs lightly. Your loved one's provider certainly isn't going to take these drugs lightly. That said, the relief that opioids can provide someone with RLS is so profound that these drugs should be considered in the proper circumstances.

Salma and Omar have been married for 2 years. Omar has been taking pramipexole for his RLS for 5 years. At a recent office visit, Omar indicated to the physician assistant caring for his RLS that

(Continued)

(Continued)

he was concerned that he was developing augmentation based on what he had read online about this problem. Having already tried iron supplementation and both gabapentin and pregabalin without relief, the physician assistant suggested he consider low-dose methadone. Omar told him that he wanted to discuss this with his wife. At home that night, Salma indicated that she was very uncomfortable with Omar taking an opioid medication because of the reports on the news about the opioid crisis. "You're not a heroin addict," she told him. "Why would you take a medication they give for heroin addiction?"

The doses of opioid medications used for RLS are very low, and they tend to stay low even after years of use. People who use opioids for RLS don't continue to increase their doses regularly. There is less risk of overdose when used as prescribed. The risks come from combining the opioid with other medications that cause sedation or with alcohol. Help keep your loved one safe by reviewing their other medications with them and their provider or their pharmacist to ensure they are safe to combine with opioids. Discourage them from consuming alcohol near the time they are taking the opioid.

The risk of developing an addiction or dependence on opioids is lower when they're used for RLS than for other conditions, but that risk still exists. Your loved one's provider will help by screening them for their risk of addiction in advance and performing urine drug screens to make sure that no other opioids besides the one(s) being prescribed are being consumed. You can assist this process by cleaning out the medicine cabinet of any old opioid prescriptions. You can also monitor for signs of an opioid addiction. The definition of an addiction is when excessive use of the drug continues despite negative personal consequences. You might notice them craving the drug, asking for their medication early, or being overly scared of running out.

If you are concerned about your loved one developing an opioid dependence or addiction, please encourage them to speak to their provider. You can also express your concerns directly to their provider. Confidentiality laws prevent providers from speaking to you without the consent of your loved one, but they are allowed to receive information from loved ones about their patients. You can also call the Substance Abuse and Mental Health Services Administration at 1-800-662-HELP (4357) to reach 24/7 substance abuse counselors who will advise you on how to get your loved one help.

Another important way to help your loved one manage their opioid medication is to keep it safe. If there are other people in your home (e.g., children, babysitters, or cleaners), encourage your loved one to keep their medication locked away. Opioid theft is real, and it is deadly. Likewise, do not take any of your loved one's opioids yourself. If you're in pain, it might be tempting to take one of their pills since they're readily available. While this is both dangerous and illegal, you probably won't die or be arrested for this, so you might think it's okay to do. It's not. Your loved one needs their medication and can only get a fixed quantity per month. This quantity is tightly regulated, and if you take some of it, they won't have enough. If they run out early or ask for a refill before it's due, they will either have to suffer until their medication is refillable or raise red flags about why they need more medicine so soon. Either outcome is bad. Please don't do this to them.

Dopamine agonists, gabapentinoids, and opioids are not the only medications that are used for RLS, but they are the most common, and they're highly effective. If your loved one has tried all of these classes of drug and has not found relief, don't give up hope. Encourage them to talk to their provider about some of the many alternatives that are less common but still viable options. It is very rare that someone has RLS that cannot be treated. It is a reasonable expectation that at least one option will be effective and tolerable, although it might take some trial and error to find it.

Advocacy

A great way to provide support to your loved one is by advocating for them. If their provider is not adequately addressing the RLS, you can attend the next appointment and speak up to reinforce how much you see your loved one suffering. You can also help by gathering resources for your loved one. The Restless Legs Syndrome Foundation, for example, is a membership organization that provides extensive information about RLS. You can join this group and find further information for patients and caregivers. Another way to advocate is through legislative advocacy for items that are important for RLS care, such as continued access to telehealth services and the ability to prescribe opioids via telehealth encounters. You can also provide financial support to institutions performing RLS research or education.

> Laurie and Pat have been married for 4 years. Laurie developed RLS when pregnant last year. It improved after delivery of their healthy baby, but now it has returned. At a routine visit with Laurie's *gynecologist*, she brought up her leg symptoms and asked what she could do about it. The gynecologist told Laurie that this was normal after pregnancy and there was nothing to be done. Pat spoke up to advocate for her, asking, "What about checking her iron levels?"

How RLS affects loved ones

You might not have RLS, but if your loved one does, you are certainly affected too. Emotionally, it is difficult to watch your loved one suffer. It is draining to be a caregiver who must provide regular reassurance, comfort, sympathy, and compassion. You might have experienced feelings of powerlessness. Hopefully, this chapter has shown you all the things you can do to help, but even that might not be enough to eliminate the discomfort they're in.

You might even have feelings of resentment if your loved one is paying more attention to their legs than to you. If you are feeling neglected by the amount of time and energy your loved one is devoting to their RLS, keep in mind, they want to be dealing with this even less than you want them to be dealing with this.

> Jamie and Jordan have been married for 11 years. They met 13 years ago in a club for people who like science fiction movies. Their tradition for years has been to watch a different sci-fi movie each Friday night. For the past year, though, Jordan has had to get up and pace around the room while they're watching. Jamie has RLS and is fairly certain that Jordan does too. Jamie has tried to convince Jordan to speak to a doctor about this, but Jordan hasn't gotten around to it yet. One Friday, Jamie snaps and yells, "I'm not going to keep watching you pace around like this. You're driving me nuts! Talk to a doctor already!"

You might not want to admit it to them, but living with a partner who has RLS can be annoying. Maybe it drives you nuts to have your loved one pacing around at night when you're trying to relax. There's something about pacing that generates feelings of anxiety in onlookers. Maybe you're sitting next to them and their leg movements are transmitted through the couch so you can feel the shaking. You know you can't blame them, but it doesn't stop you from wanting to scream, "Hold still!" If you're suffering like this, imagine how much they are.

Getting your loved one medical help is one way to help yourself. In the moment, though, you can get up and move to another seat or another room. While your loved one could be the one to move to eliminate your frustration, that shouldn't always be the solution. Sometimes, you can help by removing yourself from the situation that's bothering you. If you are getting worked up by a partner that can't hold still, just leave the room.

Have the conversation in advance when everyone is calm. Discuss the range of possible solutions for when your partner's RLS acts up. Is this a circumstance where teamwork (e.g., distraction, massage) is best, or should one of you just move to another space? The more tools you have in your toolbox to handle their discomfort and your emotions, the smoother these interactions will go, and it starts with communication.

Changing chairs or leaving the room is relatively straightforward in the evening, but sometimes the RLS symptoms don't occur until after bedtime. Have you tried sharing a bed with someone with RLS? If the leg movements while they're awake don't bother you, maybe the associated limb movements of sleep will. Bedpartners frequently complain about the periodic limb movements of sleep that are frequently seen in patients with RLS. They report that their sleep is disturbed because their loved one is jerking through the night.

Sometimes, though, periodic limb movements of sleep (PLMS) occur without underlying RLS, in which case the PLMS might be harmless (Chapter 14). That doesn't make it any less annoying for the bedpartner who lies awake counting the events or the interval of time between the events. The loved one has the diagnosis, but the bedpartner has the problem. This situation raises an ethical dilemma for the RLS provider caring for someone with PLMS. Should a patient with PLMS that bothers their bedpartner but not themselves be treated? Probably not, but this is an ambiguous situation and different providers might address this differently.

Due to RLS or PLMS, both you and your loved one with the bothersome legs might wind up sleep deprived. This is a very common complaint associated with RLS, and one of the more distressing. Everyone has experienced sleep deprivation at some point in their lives, but when it becomes a chronic, nightly problem, it can take a very high toll mentally and physically. It might become necessary to sleep in separate beds or bedrooms to protect your sleep. You don't have to suffer out of sympathy; a sleepy caregiver is just going to cause more trouble in the relationship. It's okay to take care of yourself so that you're better able to take care of your loved one.

Another one of the more common complaints by loved ones is that RLS has taken away the fun things they used to do with their partners, like traveling or going to the theater or cinema. This can be very frustrating. Airplanes, cars, and theaters have one thing in common: seats where people are confined for a long time without a lot of legroom, and these spaces are particularly difficult for people with RLS.

> Sam and Logan have been dating for a year. Sam loves to travel internationally, but ever since they started dating, they haven't traveled much because Logan is concerned about the long flights. Sam is worried about the future of their relationship if Logan can't find some way to participate in Sam's favorite activity.

Thankfully, there is hope. For people who take nightly medication for their RLS, it's usually possible to get extra doses to take before starting trips or going to shows. The as-needed booster doses can make all the difference in the world and restore your ability to do the things you love. Medications with long-term side effects, such as dopamine agonists, can be used more safely as an on-demand than as a daily medication. Encourage your loved one to ask their provider about this type of treatment if their symptoms are well controlled at night but still troublesome in specific circumstances during the day. This might be a relatively simple fix.

This is also another scenario where communication is very important. If your loved one doesn't want to travel, would they mind if you traveled without them? They might care a whole lot, in which case, you are pouring salt in the wound to leave them behind. But if travel is something that's more important to you than it is to them, they really might be happy to see you enjoying yourself. It's possible your partner feels guilty for limiting the pleasure you're getting from your life, so allowing you to enjoy the things you like to do is a way for them not to feel guilty for holding you back. Travel is just one example, of course, and this could apply to going to the theater or other sedentary events just as much.

Also consider that there might be ways to accommodate their RLS into your plans. A matinee or morning flight might be easier to tolerate than ones later in the day, for example. Could you travel to closer destinations so the flights won't be as long? Compromise isn't always the answer, but it's great when it works out well for both of you.

The only way you'll be able to work through these issues is to discuss them. Let your loved one know that you don't blame them for having a medical condition that's out of their control, while at the same time, acknowledge that it does affect you too. Let them know how you intend to help them and ask them for help in the ways that you have identified would benefit you. It's okay for you to have your own needs. It will benefit everyone if you can sort out how your family unit can work together for the most mutually satisfactory outcomes.

Summary

Being the loved one or a caregiver for someone with RLS is difficult. It's tough to watch them suffer. It's annoying to deal with the pacing and movement they might do frequently. It's draining to be sympathetic and compassionate each night. All of these emotions might be magnified if you're sleep deprived from their leg jerks keeping you awake all night.

But you are not powerless. You have a big role to play in your loved one's care, and you've taken a big step in that direction just by reading this chapter to educate yourself. Advocate for them with their health care provider. Help them track their symptoms and any triggers they might not have recognized that exacerbate their symptoms. Record their responses to medications and any side effects. Offer leg massages. If you're able, donate time or money to advance the research and care of patients with RLS. Most importantly, thank you for taking their condition seriously and for all you have done and will do to make your loved one's life with RLS better.

CHAPTER 17

Unanswered Questions and the Future of RLS Management

In this chapter, you will learn:

- What aspects of RLS remain unexplained
- What might the future hold for the diagnosis and treatment of RLS

Introduction

With all that is known about RLS, there's even more that is unknown. There are still uncertainties at every stage: what causes RLS, how best to diagnose it, what the best treatment strategy is, and so on. This chapter will review the unanswered questions about RLS and what, if anything, is being done to answer them. It will also gaze into the near future and speculate where the world of RLS care might be headed.

Causes of RLS

Genetics

Starting at the most fundamental level, it's not clear just how big of a role your genes might play in RLS. We know that some genes predispose you to RLS, but not everyone with an RLS-related gene has RLS, and not everyone with RLS has one of these genes. Maybe people who don't have one of the known RLS genes have a currently unknown RLS gene. Or maybe they have RLS that is unrelated to their genetics. It's likely that there are RLS-causing genes that haven't been discovered yet. The field of genome sequencing is still rapidly evolving, and much is being learned about how genes are turned on and off based on your environment. Putting all of this together for RLS will take many years, but if we can sort out the genetics of RLS, we will learn much about the changes in the brain that are responsible for the symptoms.

The current hypothesis is that not everyone with RLS has a genetic cause. This makes it even trickier to pin down why you developed symptoms. Iron deficiency in the brain is a well-known source of RLS, but why do some people develop low brain iron when their blood iron levels are fine? Genetics would be one answer, but are there other possibilities? There are hormones that regulate iron in the blood. There are likely hormones that regulate iron passage into the brain, but which ones and how they work is not well known. Could we find a way to open the blood-brain barrier and let more iron in? The process of iron regulation in the brain is still an active area of research. Understanding how to better get iron into the brain could be a significant therapeutic advance in RLS therapy.

Inflammation

Inflammation in the body, which is the body's chemical response to disease or stress, is known to worsen RLS, but how and why this happens is unknown. It is possible that inflammation controls how much iron gets into your brain. Over time, **chronic inflammation** could worsen RLS by exacerbating a brain iron deficiency. This could explain why there are associations between RLS and autoimmune diseases, such as **Crohn's disease**, and other medical conditions, such as **small intestinal bacterial overgrowth (SIBO)**, that are associated with high inflammation. On the other hand, some research has shown that inflammation can increase iron in the brain, so more studies are needed to sort out the relationship between chronic inflammation and brain iron.

The abrupt worsening of symptoms at times of **acute inflammation** is too sudden to attribute to iron changes, though. It is hard to imagine that contracting COVID-19 or having surgery changes the iron levels in your brain enough to trigger RLS. Something else about inflammation must be responsible for this exacerbation. What makes this so tricky is that inflammation is not a single entity; inflammation is a constellation of changes that occur via the body's immune system, so understanding which inflammatory compounds in the blood are the ones responsible for RLS would be a major advance in our understanding. Unlocking the secrets of the body's inflammatory responses could improve care for RLS and many other diseases as well.

Neurotransmitters

One of the great aspects of science is that it changes direction as more is learned. For many years, insufficient dopamine production was thought to cause RLS. It turns out that this is probably not true. Add to that the relatively recent discoveries that glutamate and adenosine abnormalities play a role in RLS, and the entire paradigm for understanding RLS has changed. The next step is to put all of these pieces together. There are theories as to how these pathways interact, but the complexity of the brain essentially guarantees that our current understanding is still overly simplistic. For example, serotonin is almost certainly involved in RLS given that drugs that increase serotonin often exacerbate restlessness, but exactly what serotonin does and how it interacts with the other neurotransmitters to cause RLS are unknown.

Opioid medications are among the most effective treatments for RLS, but what is not understood is *why* they are so effective. Your brain naturally makes opioids that function as neurotransmitters, and how those are involved in generating RLS is another open question.

Naturally occurring opioids in the brain likely interact with the dopamine pathways. There are still many details of this interaction that need elucidating. Research in mice is ongoing to try to answer these questions.

Melatonin, a brain hormone, also plays an as yet undefined role in RLS. Melatonin regulates the **circadian rhythm**, and RLS is a **circadian disorder**, meaning that it gets worse at night and better during the day. Some people who take melatonin supplements find their RLS worsens, presumably through the same mechanism that causes RLS to naturally worsen later in the day. Melatonin regulates multiple neurotransmitters, including reducing dopamine, so this seems to be how it could affect RLS, but the details still need to be sorted out.

Most of the numerous neurotransmitters in the brain have never been studied for a possible role in RLS. The brain is a hugely complex system, and we are only scratching the surface of all the chemical changes that come together to cause RLS. To make it even more complicated, each person could have a different set of changes, maybe with only one element in common that leads to the similar sensations people often describe. Understanding the causes of RLS is one of the best ways to develop new therapies, or—if we dare to dream—a cure.

Anatomy

Anatomically, no fewer than 13 different regions of the brain have been studied for their role in causing RLS. There are target areas that seem to be more relevant than others, but this only reinforces how complex RLS is likely to be, and how our current models are probably inadequate. With all this attention on the brain, though, the nerves and blood supply to the legs themselves are often overlooked.

Among RLS experts, it is still debated if the legs have a role in the cause of RLS. At this time, other than identifying a peripheral neuropathy, your RLS provider is not likely to spend much time talking about or evaluating your legs, which is ironic given that your legs are most likely the site of your discomfort. However, there is reason to believe that blood flow into and out of the legs might contribute to RLS. Health care providers might be missing a large group of patients who would benefit from more directed therapy by not looking at the **arteries** and **veins** in the legs. We simply don't understand all the ways in which the legs are involved—if they are at all—in causing RLS symptoms.

Diagnosing RLS

The current diagnostic approach to RLS is subjective. If your symptoms match what the textbooks say (an urge to move your legs that is worse at rest, is worse in the evening, improves with movement, and has no better explanation than RLS), the diagnosis is straightforward. But bodies don't read textbooks, and there are cases of RLS that are not as obvious. These criteria might be overly restrictive and miss people who have RLS. They might be overly inclusive and lead to false diagnoses of RLS. It would be helpful in these situations to have an objective test for RLS.

There is no MRI or **CT scan** of the brain that will confirm an RLS diagnosis. However, there are advanced tests based on MRI technology or radioactivity that could potentially be harnessed for RLS testing in the future. **Dopamine transporter (DaT) scans** use radioactivity to identify dopamine in the brain. These are currently used to evaluate for Parkinson's disease, a condition in which dopamine stops being produced, but given dopamine's role in RLS, a similar technique might be developed for RLS in the future.

While a traditional MRI looks at the structure of the brain, two other MRI techniques, **functional MRI (fMRI)** and **MR spectroscopy**, have already been used to help better understand the brains of people with RLS. fMRI relies on changes in blood flow to different regions of the brain to create pictures of what regions of the brain are most active over time. MR spectroscopy uses properties of magnetism to determine which chemicals are most prevalent in different areas of the brain at a given moment. While neither of these techniques is used for diagnosing RLS currently, it's possible to envision a world where specific fMRI or MR spectroscopy findings can tell us who is likely to have RLS.

One area where brain imaging is already being used diagnostically for RLS is in identifying brain iron deficiency using ultrasound. Your RLS can't be diagnosed this way, but it can tell you what your brain iron status is. Being able to better determine who has brain iron deficiency and who would most benefit from supplemental iron therapy would be a monumental advance in the care of people with RLS. There are several benefits of brain ultrasounds. First, they can monitor iron levels directly in the brain, rather than relying on blood tests or spinal fluid analysis from a spinal tap. Blood tests are easier to perform than spinal fluid analysis, but even blood tests require needles. Ultrasounds are less invasive than a blood test, and the result is more relevant. Second, ultrasound is safe. There is no medical limit to the number of ultrasounds you can receive, which means your iron levels can be tracked over time without any risk to you. Third, this can be done in the clinic without any special preparation on your part.

The two major hurdles to the wider use of ultrasound in the care of RLS are a lack of training to perform this procedure among American RLS providers and a lack of reimbursement by insurance companies for doing it. Nevertheless, given the advantages, it seems likely that over time, this will become more commonly performed. It should be noted that MRIs can assess for brain iron also, but this is much more costly and time consuming than an ultrasound, and the technique for using MRIs for brain iron assessment in RLS is not as well defined.

We will continue to rely on blood iron tests until ultrasound becomes available. The optimal way to interpret iron studies is still debated, though. Are the current thresholds of 75 µg/L of ferritin and a transferrin saturation of 20% the best levels to use? Many RLS experts think these numbers are too low. The common practice currently is to test for iron and treat with supplements if the levels are deemed to be too low. In the future, this could shift to checking iron levels and treating everyone who is not deemed to be too high (ferritin higher than 300 µg/L and transferrin saturation above 45%). This would lead to much more iron therapy than is currently performed. It would likely help the many patients with iron levels above the current threshold to treat who are nevertheless brain iron deficient.

Other than the current practice of checking iron levels in the blood for everyone with RLS, there are no routinely performed tests. This could change in the future, though. Vitamin D deficiency has been associated with RLS and is very straightforward to correct, so checking vitamin D levels might become a standard of care in the future. Over time, other blood tests might be discovered that would be relevant as well. Likewise, nerve tests and blood flow tests of the legs might become more commonplace in the care of people with RLS as we learn more about causes of RLS outside the brain.

The future of RLS treatment

Despite its critical role in treating RLS, iron supplementation is not currently considered first-line therapy in the medical guidelines. Iron is advised as an addition to other therapies. This is certain to change. Iron, particularly intravenous iron, is simply too effective and too safe not to pursue. Many RLS providers already practice this way, but the guidelines have not yet caught up.

After iron therapy, what's next? For many years, the answer has been dopamine agonists. This too must change. The odds of developing tolerance, augmentation, an impulse control disorder, or some combination of these are too high to justify using these drugs as first-line therapies (Chapter 7). Most likely, the answer will be gabapentinoids. While these drugs have their downsides too, they have less potential for harm than the dopamine agonists. Most importantly, you do not get worse the longer you take them.

The order in which you try medications might make a difference also. Does taking a dopamine agonist first put you at a disadvantage for successful treatment with a gabapentinoid in the future? Does taking a gabapentinoid make dopamine agonists more or less effective? Does the order in which you are exposed to them change the risk of complications? It's not known if long-term exposure to these drugs causes any changes in the brain that would make it important to start with one or the other first. The only sequence that is known to be important is treating iron deficiency prior to starting dopamine agonists because iron deficiency can predispose you to having augmentation or impulse control disorders in the setting of these medications.

In an ideal world, providers would know in advance which medications you are likely to tolerate well and respond to symptomatically. This is called precision medicine, and it would be much better than the current practice of trial and error to find you the right medication. For some types of medications, such as antidepressants, this type of approach is already gaining steam. You can have a blood test done that will predict which antidepressants you should try and which you should avoid based on genetic factors. No such test exists for RLS, but maybe someday it will.

Aside from the four major classes of RLS medication (dopamine agonists, gabapentinoids, opioids, and benzodiazepines), Chapter 11 discussed many other options for treatment. Over time, more research will hopefully elucidate which of these should be utilized more frequently. Maybe one of them will someday replace gabapentinoids as the preferred first-line medication. Understanding the neurological pathways that lead to RLS will facilitate this type of drug discovery. For example, when it was discovered that changes in adenosine were contributing to RLS, a trial of dipyridamole, a drug that increases adenosine activity, was tested for RLS and found to be effective. Maybe drugs that affect serotonin, histamine, or melatonin will be harnessed for RLS in the future.

Augmentation from dopamine agonists is an awful complication of therapy. If a dopamine-related medication could be designed that did not lead to this outcome, we might be able to get the beneficial effects of dopamine therapy without this disastrous consequence. For now, though, designing the optimal treatment for people who suffer from augmentation is a goal for the future.

While several protocols exist for helping you stop a dopamine agonist, it's not known which one is best in the long run. And does it help to get you off the medication faster? Maybe that will help jump start your recovery. Or is the faster taper of the medication just going to cause you more suffering while a slower approach would cushion your withdrawal symptoms? Some RLS providers will use another medication, such as a gabapentinoid or opioid, to help you stop your dopamine agonist, but there is no set protocol to tell providers which drug and which dose is best for this purpose.

It's important to remember that not all therapy comes in the form of a pill. There are many nonpharmacological options for RLS (Chapter 6), but there are no protocols or guidelines for how to integrate these into your care. A healthy diet and regular exercise might go a long way to treating RLS. Therapies that are currently experimental, such as infrared light and lasers, might one day become standard therapy. As helpful as medications can be, most people would choose to avoid a drug if an alternative approach were equally effective, so more research is needed on the best ways to treat RLS without drugs.

Research

There is still a tremendous amount to learn about RLS. While some of the work on understanding RLS will be done by scientists in laboratories, you can help advance the field of RLS yourself. Researchers will need people with RLS to participate in their research. This might involve providing blood or spinal fluid samples, undergoing brain imaging tests like ultrasounds or MRIs, having nerve or blood flow tests, or any number of other possibilities. This could also involve taking medications as part of a drug research study to find new treatments for RLS. Knowledge of RLS can only advance with the help of those of you who have the condition. Your loved ones can help too. Many of these research studies will need people without RLS for comparison. If you have the chance to participate in RLS research, I hope you will do so. Your contribution could change many lives.

Final thoughts

I am truly sorry that you have to live with this miserable condition. Some of you are dealing with intense suffering, possibly exacerbated by the medications you were prescribed. The most important messages I hope you take from this book are:

1. **You do not need to suffer forever.** There are effective treatments!
2. **Your suffering deserves to be taken seriously.** No matter what else you're dealing with, RLS should not be ignored.
3. **Iron is critical.** Start by addressing iron levels and everything else follows from there.
4. **Dopamine agonists are far more dangerous and addictive than people think.** There are safe ways to use these effective drugs, but daily consumption of high doses is not the answer.
5. **There is still much to learn about RLS.** As much as we think we know, there's even more still to be discovered.

ACKNOWLEDGMENTS

Dr. Andy Berkowski, my RLS brother. Meeting Andy was like looking in a mirror, and not just because of our name. No one I know is more aligned to my way of thinking about RLS. He introduced me to the International Restless Legs Syndrome Study Group, where I found other like-minded colleagues. I've truly enjoyed talking about RLS with Andy, bouncing ideas off him, and asking him questions. He's a true expert. You've got next, Andy.

Dr. Charlene Gamaldo, the epitome of sponsorship. I am forever indebted to you for the support you've shown me during my career. A renowned RLS expert in her own right, Dr. Gamaldo is an amazing leader and trailblazer. It's an honor to consider her a colleague and friend.

Dr. Doug Kirsch, mentor, sponsor. Doug is a distinguished leader in the field of sleep medicine, and I aspire to the heights he has reached. Doug has done so much for me over the course of my career, I probably don't know half of it because he won't admit it. It's been a tremendous honor moving from his student to his friend.

Prof. Mitch Prinstein, my role model. Seeing you writing your book week in and week out gave me the courage to try writing one myself. You showed me that doing anything is possible, and you showed me that doing everything is possible.

Dr. Sanford Auerbach, my sleep medicine fellowship program director at Boston Medical Center. So much of who I am as a sleep doctor comes from Dr. Auerbach. Formal sleep medicine training only lasts 1 year, and he packed me full of as much knowledge as he could and set me up for success.

My colleagues at Duke, especially those who practice sleep medicine: Dr. Aatif Husain; Dr. Rod Radtke; Dr. Ann Augustine; Dr. Maggie Soltis; Dr. Wissam Mansour; Dr. Shalu Bansal; Dr. Mariam Wasim; Dr. Sushrusha Arjyal; Irene Abella, DNP; Kelly Blessing, FNP; Susannah White, PA-C; Alisa Wilczynski, PA-C; Caitlyn Gallagher, FNP, and Steve Taxman, PA-C, along with the teams at the Duke Sleep Disorders Center and Duke Neurology South Durham. You have challenged me, encouraged me, questioned me, taught me, vented with me, and, most of all, provided outstanding care to all our patients. And to the chair of Duke Neurology Dr. Rich O'Brien, who is my biggest cheerleader and advocate, always supporting my changing ideas for what I want from my career. Finally, to my former Duke colleague Dr. Alan Tesson, who shares my interest in finding new ways to treat RLS without medications.

Craig Panner from Oxford University Press, a phenomenal editor and guide. Craig gave me the confidence that I could write a whole book and guided me every step of the way. I now have a new friend to see at our annual neurology and sleep medicine conferences. This book does not happen without Craig.

Ilse Irving, AP English teacher, Garber High School, Essexville, MI. It has been over 25 years since I took her class, and if anyone had told me at the time that I would one day write a book, I would've laughed at them. Mrs. Irving gave me the writing foundation that would carry me through the rest of my education and career. I had no idea at the time that being a physician required writing skills, but it absolutely does, and I'm sure glad I paid attention and had a master educator to prepare me.

Kathy Kinkema and Samantha Shad, who graciously agreed to provide the patient perspective in reviewing this manuscript. Their insights into how this book would be viewed by the target audience were invaluable.

Keosha Brumant, our nanny extraordinaire. Keosha has been with the family for years, which means she saw us through the COVID-19 pandemic. When schools closed, she jumped into action and created her own home school to keep my kids educated. With two busy physicians for parents, having her help has given me the mental capacity and time to work on this book. Having someone you completely trust with your children is one of life's biggest blessings.

Jill Lipman, my aunt. When she heard I was writing a book about RLS, I soon received a packet in the mail of information about procedures to replace medications for RLS. This information was incorporated into Chapter 6.

Joel and Nicole Spector, my brother and sister-in-law. I am counting on you to help me promote this book as you travel the world! Maybe now I'll have more time to join some of your adventures.

The Iweala family, my in-laws. From day 1, you've made me part of your family, but authoring a book seems like a real rite of passage to be a full member. If the busiest person I know could write several books, I had no excuse. Thank you for the unconditional love and support. Uzo, thanks for helping me across the finish line.

Kayla and Arthur Spector, my parents. Although I'm fairly sure my mother thought I was crazy for agreeing to write a book, my parents consistently encouraged me and supported me, convincing me that I could do whatever I put my mind to. It's cliché, but they really did say that. I think I'll be most proud of the moment I can put a copy of this book in their hands.

Adaora, Emeka, and Kelechi, my children. You are amazing, loving, kind, and generous. You never complained about my spending weekend mornings writing. You are very cooperative and get to bed on time, which is one of the best gifts a child can give a dad who is a sleep doctor. I don't know if any of you will ever write a book, but if you ever wonder if you can, know that I have no doubt. I love you all so much! And to Adaora, whose creative talents generated the figures for this book, I am incredibly grateful!

Onyi, my wife. You have certainly put up with a lot of talk about RLS and this book. I promise you no more talk about page counts, unfinished chapters, or my general stress about staying on deadline anymore. Thank you for letting me bounce ideas off you, write side by side with you, and vent to you. You never once questioned my sanity for agreeing to add on this project to everything else I was already doing. If ever a spouse were a true partner, it's you.

TREATMENT ALGORITHM

Below you will find a sample treatment algorithm for RLS. Every patient is different, and this is not meant to tell you what you should do. All treatments must be discussed with health care providers who know the details of your medical history. This is simply meant as an example of a common approach to treating RLS.

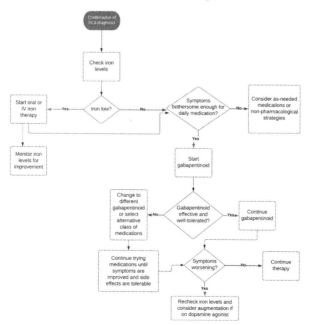

.

GLOSSARY

Abuse: The improper or excessive use of potentially harmful drugs or substances.

Acetaminophen: A medication used for reducing pain and fever.

Acupuncture: A component of Traditional Chinese Medicine that involves inserting small needles into the body at specific points.

Acute inflammation: short-term activation of the immune system.

Adenosine: In the context of sleep, adenosine is a compound found in the brain that signals sleepiness as it increases; derangements in adenosine signals have been implicated in RLS.

Adrenal gland: An organ located near the kidneys that secretes cortisol.

Agonist: A substance that stimulates increased response by a neuron, typically enhancing, mimicking, or replacing the action of a naturally occurring substance. Agonists are the opposite of antagonists, which block or reduce normal functioning.

Air hunger: An unpleasant sensation marked by a feeling of being unable to take in enough air; a form of shortness of breath.

Akathisia: The medical term used to describe difficulty holding still.

Alpha-2-delta ligands: See gabapentinoids.

Alpha-2-delta receptors: The targets for gabapentinoid medications.

Antidepressants: A class of medications that treat depression and anxiety; they are sometimes used for various other medical conditions as well.

Antihistamine: A category of medicine that blocks histamine, often used to reduce allergic symptoms or stomach acid.

Antinausea: A category of medicine that reduces the sense of nausea.

Antipsychotic: A category of medicine that reduces the symptoms of psychosis, such as hallucinations and delusions.

Anxiety: An unpleasant sensation of fear or dread.

Arteries: Tubes for moving blood away from the heart.

Asterixis: Sudden, brief, recurrent loss of muscle tone, frequently assessed by extending the arms and hands as if pushing on a wall and watching for a flapping effect.

Attention deficit hyperactivity disorder: A condition that typically manifests in childhood, characterized by inattention, hyperactivity, or impulsivity.

Augmentation: The worsening of RLS symptoms due to the medications used to treat it, most often dopamine agonists. This manifests as symptoms starting sooner after becoming sedentary, starting earlier in the day, affecting additional body parts (e.g., arms), or having a longer delay between medication administration and relief of symptoms.

Autoimmune diseases: A group of diseases in which a person's immune system attacks their own healthy tissues.

Autonomic: Functions of the body that do not require thought or intention, such as breathing, digestion, heart rate, blood pressure control, and sweating.

Benzodiazepine use disorder: A physical or psychological dependence on benzodiazepine medications with continued use despite known harm.

Benzodiazepines: A class of drugs that reduce brain activity as a means of treating conditions such as seizures, anxiety, and insomnia.

Benzos: A nickname for benzodiazepines.

Biopsy: A diagnostic test performed by removing a small sample from the body.

Black box warning: The strongest level of warning issued by the US Food and Drug Administration about a medication.

Blood-brain barrier: A network of structures that restrict the types of substances that can pass from the blood into the brain.

Blood protein: A nonspecific term that refers to molecules composed of amino acids that circulate in the blood.

Blood vessels: Arteries and veins that move blood around the body.

Brain iron deficiency: Inadequate levels of iron in the brain.

Bromocriptine: A medication in the dopamine agonist class, previously used to treat RLS.

Cannabidiol (CBD): One of many chemicals found in the cannabis sativa plant, commonly marketed for a variety of medicinal purposes.

Cannabis: Also known as marijuana, it is a plant that contains numerous psychoactive and nonpsychoactive chemicals.

Carbidopa/levodopa: A combination of two medications that functions as supplemental dopamine, frequently used to treat Parkinson's disease and previously RLS.

Central sleep apnea: Recurrent episodes of breathing pauses while sleeping not due to an obstruction in the airway often associated with heart or brain diseases or certain medications.

Chelated iron: A form of nonheme oral iron supplement.

Chronic inflammation: Long-term activation of the immune system.

Circadian disorder: Any of several conditions that impair the sleep-wake cycle due to abnormalities in the circadian rhythm.

Circadian rhythm: Body processes that follow an approximately 24-hour cycle.

Classical conditioning: A phenomenon in which learning occurs without conscious effort by repeatedly pairing something neutral with something that elicits a reaction.

Clinical diagnosis: A method making a diagnosis using a history and physical exam rather than laboratory, imaging, or other tests.

Clinical trial: A type of research to determine the effectiveness of a medical intervention.

Cognitive: A term that refers generally to various types of thinking and mental processing.

Cognitive behavioral therapy for insomnia: First-line therapy to help improve sleep using strategies to change thoughts and behaviors around sleep.

Colonoscopy: A medical procedure that utilizes a fiberoptic camera to visualize the inside of the colon (large intestine).

Coma: A prolonged state of unconsciousness typically caused by a brain injury or medication.

Compression stockings: A type of sock that squeezes the legs.

Continuous positive airway pressure (CPAP) machine : A device that uses air pressure to help prevent the airway from collapsing, used to treat obstructive sleep apnea.

Controlled substance: A medication that is considered worthy of increased regulation by the Drug Enforcement Agency due to greater associated risks.

Copay: A cost-sharing strategy used by insurance companies that assigns a fixed payment to the patient to access health care services and medications.

Coronary artery disease: Blockages in the blood vessels that supply blood to the heart.

Correlation without causation: The principle by which two things can be related without one necessarily causing the other.

Corticosteroids: A class of medication that reduces allergic responses and inflammation. Also, a class of naturally occurring hormones produced by the adrenal gland.

Cortisol: A hormone produced by the adrenal gland that increases during stress.

Counterstimulation: A technique of treating RLS that relies on distracting the brain with alternative sensations.

COVID-19: Abbreviation for coronavirus disease of 2019; an illness caused by the SARS-CoV-2 virus.

Crohn's disease: An autoimmune disease of the digestive tract, most commonly the intestines; an inflammatory bowel disease.

CT scan: Computerized tomography scan; a way of taking detailed images of the body using x-rays.

Cystic fibrosis: A genetic disease that affects the lungs and other organs.

Dementia: A nonspecific, acquired class of conditions in which a person's daily functioning is impaired due to cognitive dysfunction.

Dependence: The continued use of drugs or substances despite physical, social, or emotional harm or the desire to stop.

Depression: A mood marked by feeling sad, feeling hopeless, or losing interest in activities.

Diabetes: Short for diabetes mellitus, a condition in which blood sugar is abnormally high.

Dialysis: A medical procedure that filters the blood that is utilized when kidneys can no longer adequately do so.

Diaphragm: The primary muscle that controls breathing; when it contracts, air fills the lungs.

Diuretics: Drugs that increase the volume of urine to remove fluid from the body.

Diversion: The abuse or illegal redistribution of prescription medications.

Dopamine: A chemical messenger in the brain that plays a variety of roles, including controlling movement, reward, and hallucinations. Derangements in dopamine have been associated with RLS.

Dopamine agonist withdrawal syndrome: A collection of severe symptoms that affects some people who discontinue use of dopamine agonists, typically manifesting with anxiety, depression, fatigue, body pain, or low blood pressure and lightheadedness when standing up.

Dopamine transporter (DaT) scans: An imaging procedure that involves injecting a radioactive tracer that attaches to the dopamine transporter in the brain to determine the functioning of dopamine, most commonly used to aid in the diagnosis of Parkinson's disease.

Dysesthesia: The medical term for abnormal sensations in the body, usually used in reference to something unpleasant.

Electrocardiogram: Also known as an ECG or EKG, this is a diagnostic test of the electrical functioning of the heart.

Electromyogram (EMG): A diagnostic test performed by recording the electrical activity in a muscle, typically using a small needle inserted into the muscle. This test is used to assess for nerve and muscle diseases.

Elemental iron: The component of an iron supplement that is pure iron, used to compare the amount of iron in different types of iron supplements.

Embryonic: A term that refers to the first 10 weeks of development of human offspring.

Epilepsy: A brain disorder characterized by abnormalities of the electrical circuits of the brain resulting in seizures.

Estrogen: The primary hormone responsible for generating female sexual characteristics.

Excitatory: Something that increases the rate at which a neuron will transmit signals.

Fatigue: Tiredness, lack of energy.

Ferric carboxymaltose : An intravenous iron product that can be used for RLS.

Ferric citrate : A form of nonheme oral iron supplement.

Ferric sulfate: A form of nonheme oral iron supplement.

Ferritin: A protein found in the blood that stores iron.

Ferrous fumarate: A form of nonheme oral iron supplement.

Ferrous gluconate: A form of nonheme oral iron supplement.

Ferrous sulfate: The most commonly recommended form of nonheme oral iron supplement.

Ferumoxytol: An intravenous iron product that can be used for RLS.

Fetal: A term that refers to the development of offspring after the first 10 weeks until birth.

Fibromyalgia: A chronic pain condition characterized by pain throughout the body, low energy, and trouble sleeping, thought to be due to changes in how the brain processes sensory information from the body.

Folate: One of the B vitamins (B_9) that is necessary for health and is especially critical to healthy pregnancies.

Folic acid: A synthetic form of folate (vitamin B_9) that can be used to increase folate levels in the body.

Functional MRI (fMRI): An MRI technique that allows an assessment of which areas of the brain are active over time, relying on the concept that more active areas of the brain receive more blood supply.

GABA (gamma-aminobutyric acid): A neurotransmitter that is responsible for reducing the actions of other neurons.

Gabapentin: A medication in the gabapentinoid class, frequently used to treat RLS and other conditions.

Gabapentin enacarbil: A medication in the gabapentinoid class that is approved to treat RLS.

Gabapentinoids: A class of medications that includes gabapentin, pregabalin, and gabapentin enacarbil. These drugs have numerous clinical uses.

Gastroparesis: A condition in which the food moves excessively slowly through the digestive tract.

Generalized anxiety disorder: A condition characterized by excessive worry about multiple, everyday occurrences.

Generic: A version of a medication sold after the expiration of a patent on the brand-name medication.

Genes: A unit of DNA that transmits traits between parents and children.

Genetic: Relating to genes, which are units of DNA that transmit traits between parents and children.

Gestational: A term that refers to something that happens during pregnancy.

Glia: Cells in the brain other than neurons that are responsible for maintaining the optimal environment for neurons to function.

Gynecologist: A physician who specializes in care of the female reproductive system.

Half-life: The amount of time it takes for the concentration of a drug in the body to decrease by half.

Hallucinations: The perception of something that is not really present. These can affect any sense (e.g., hearing, vision, taste, smell, touch).

Heart failure: A condition in which the heart's ability to pump blood cannot meet the demand of the body.

Hematologist: A physician who treats diseases of the blood.

Heme iron: Iron derived from animal sources that is more readily absorbed by the body than nonheme iron.

Hemochromatosis: A disease characterized by abnormal processing of iron in the body leading to excessive iron in the blood or body tissues. People with this condition should not be treated with iron supplements or infusions.

High-molecular-weight iron dextran: An intravenous iron product that is no longer available due to the high rate of allergic reactions.

Hormone: A chemical messenger transmitted through the bloodstream.

Hypnic jerks: Also known as sleep starts and hypnagogic jerks, these are sudden, brief jerking movements that occur just prior to falling asleep.

Impulse control disorder: The inability to suppress the urge to perform certain behaviors; a possible complication of dopamine agonist medications. These most often manifest as compulsive eating, shopping, gambling, or sexual behaviors.

In utero: A term that refers to something that takes place while offspring are still in the uterus (i.e., prior to birth).

Inattention: Difficulty paying attention and easily distracted.

Inhibitory: Something that decreases the rate at which a neuron will transmit signals.

Insomnia: Difficulty falling or staying asleep or waking up too early despite the opportunity to sleep.

Intravenously: Medications administered directly into the bloodstream through a vein.

Iron deficiency: Inadequate levels of iron in the blood or brain.

Iron gluconate: A form on intravenous iron not typically used for RLS.

Iron infusion reaction: A minor reaction to receiving an infusion of intravenous iron that consists of flushing, chest tightness, and itching but without signs of an allergic reaction, such as shortness of breath, wheezing, swelling, or changes in blood pressure.

Iron isomaltoside: An intravenous iron product that can be used for RLS.

Iron sucrose: A form on intravenous iron not typically used for RLS.

Kidney disease: A reduction in the ability of the kidneys to filter blood.

Large-fiber nerves: Specialized nerves that are responsible for transmitting signals from the brain and spinal cord to the muscles to cause movement or to transmit signals from the body to the brain regarding pressure or vibration sensations and the position of the body.

Large-fiber neuropathy: Damaged or disordered large-fiber nerves.

Limb movement arousal: A disturbance in sleep due to muscle activity in one or more limbs.

Long COVID: A poorly understood collection of symptoms that persist following resolution of acute COVID-19.

Long QT syndrome: A heart condition in which the electrical signals of the heart are abnormally conducted, leading to a higher risk of cardiac arrest.

Low blood pressure: A blood pressure that is insufficient to provide adequate blood flow to the brain and body or a pressure below 90/60 mm Hg in an adult.

Low-molecular-weight iron dextran: An intravenous iron product that can be used for RLS.

Magnesium: An element used by the body in numerous chemical reactions, sold as a dietary supplement.

Magnetic resonance imaging (MRI): A way of taking detailed images of the body using the properties of magnets.

Marijuana: See cannabis.

Mast cell activation syndrome: An immune system disorder characterized by recurrent episodes of severe allergic reactions called anaphylaxis.

Melatonin: A hormone made in the brain that regulates the body's internal clock.

Migraine: A brain disorder most frequently characterized by recurrent, severe headaches.

MR spectroscopy: An MRI technique that allows for the identification of different chemicals in specified locations in the brain.

Multiple chemical sensitivity: A disorder characterized by illness due to exposure to a wide array of substances, such as those found commonly in the environment.

Multiple sclerosis: A disease of the brain and spinal cord due to damage caused by the body's own immune system.

Myoclonus: The medical term for a sudden, brief jerking movement.

Narcolepsy: A brain disease that causes severe daytime sleepiness and other sleep-related symptoms.

Narcotics: See opioids.

Near-infrared light therapy: A technique used to treat RLS and other conditions that relies on light that is outside the visual spectrum.

Nerve: A bundle of fibers that send electrical impulses throughout the body.

Nerve conduction study: A diagnostic test performed to assess the function of nerves by applying an electric shock to one end of a nerve and measuring the response at the other end of the nerve. This test is used to diagnose nerve damage.

Neurologist: A physician who cares for disorders of the brain, spinal cord, nerves, and muscles.

Neuron: A cell that transmits electrical information through the nervous system.

Neurotransmitter: A category of chemicals that communicate messages in the nervous system.

Nocturnal dip: A phenomenon in which the blood pressure drops overnight while sleeping.

Nonheme iron: Iron derived from plant sources that is less readily absorbed by the body than heme iron.

Norepinephrine: A chemical messenger in the brain and a hormone made by the adrenal gland that is increased in times of stress or arousal.

Obesity: Excessive body fat.

Obstetrician: A physician who specializes in medical care related to pregnancy and childbirth.

Obstructive sleep apnea: Also known as OSA, a disease characterized by recurrent collapse of the airway leading to blockages and impaired breathing while asleep.

Off-label: Any use of a medication for a purpose other than what it was approved for by the US Food and Drug Administration.

Opiates: Naturally occurring substances related to opium.

Opioid: A class of drugs derived from opium with pain-relieving properties.

Opioid Risk Tool : A questionnaire used to predict the likelihood of developing opioid dependence.

Opioid use disorder: A physical or psychological dependence on opioid medications with continued use despite known harm.

Opium: A highly addictive drug derived from a specific poppy and used to generate euphoria or pain relief.

Orally: Mediations administered by mouth.

Oxycodone: A commonly prescribed opioid medication.

Painful legs moving toes syndrome: A rare medical condition defined by pain in the lower legs and toes that move involuntarily.

Pandemic: A large-scale outbreak of a disease that affects a whole country or the world.

Panic attacks: A sudden sensation of intense anxiety or dread, out of proportion to any actual danger.

Panic disorder: A condition characterized by recurrent panic attacks, which are brief, sudden, and intense episodes of anxiety and a sense of panic.

Parkinson's disease: A degenerative brain disease characterized by slow movement, tremor, walking difficulty, and stiff muscles. It is associated with loss of dopamine-producing neurons.

Pergolide: A medication in the dopamine agonist class, previously used to treat RLS. Currently off the market due to safety concerns.

Periodic limb movement disorder (PLMD): A condition in which periodic limb movements of sleep disrupt sleep enough to cause daytime symptoms, such as sleepiness.

Periodic limb movement (PLM) index: The frequency of periodic limb movements of sleep, calculated dividing the total number of periodic limb movements of sleep by the number of hours of sleep.

Periodic limb movements of sleep (PLMS): Spontaneous, jerking movements of the legs, arms, or both that occur at semiregular intervals while asleep.

Periodic limb movements of wake (PLMW): Spontaneous, jerking movements of the legs, arms, or both that occur at semiregular intervals while sedentary.

Peripheral edema: Swelling, particularly in the legs, caused by fluid accumulation.

Peripheral nervous system: The elements of the nervous system outside the brain and spinal cord, predominantly consisting of nerves and muscles.

Peripheral neuropathy: Damaged or disordered nerves. There are many different causes of peripheral neuropathy. Common symptoms include numbness, pain, or weakness, most frequently affecting the feet or hands.

Peroneal nerve: A nerve in the lower leg that is the target of a stimulation device to treat RLS.

Physician assistant: A licensed health care provider who works alongside physicians and nurse practitioners to provide medical care in many medical settings.

Placebo: An inert substance meant to mimic an active substance.

Pneumatic compression device: A machine that squeezes the legs.

Polysomnography (PSG): Also known as a sleep study, this is a test of multiple parameters during sleep, including brain waves, heart rate, breathing, and leg movements, that is performed in a sleep lab.

Potency: The degree of response from a given dose of a drug; higher-potency drugs require lower doses to be effective.

Pramipexole: A medication in the dopamine agonist class, frequently used to treat RLS and Parkinson's disease.

Pregabalin: A medication in the gabapentinoid class, frequently used to treat RLS and other conditions.

Premedication: Medication given prior to an infusion to reduce the risk of allergic reactions or side effects from the infused medication.

Prenatal vitamins: A multivitamin specifically formulated to improve the chances of a healthy pregnancy.

Prevalence: The percentage of the population that has a particular condition.

Prior authorization: A process of additional paperwork and bureaucratic hurdles used by insurance companies to increase their ability to delay or deny paying for care.

Progesterone: A hormone that prepares and supports the female reproduction system during pregnancy.

Prolactin: The hormone responsible for breast growth and milk production.

Proprietary blends: A term for commercial products that combine multiple substances in ratios that are not divulged.

Psychiatric: Relating to psychiatry, the medical field devoted to mental health care.

QT interval: A measurement of electrical signals in the heart.

Rebound: The intense recurrence of symptoms when the effect of a medication wears off.

Receptors: The part of a neuron responsible for receiving chemical messages.

Refractory: Symptoms that do not respond to multiple medications.

Relapse: The resumption of drug use after a period of sobriety.

Repetitive transcranial magnetic stimulation (rTMS): A procedure that uses magnets to stimulate the brain.

Respiratory depression: A reduction in the brain's drive to trigger breathing.

Restiffic: A commercial product that wraps around the foot and provides stimulation to reduce the sensation of RLS.

Restless legs syndrome (RLS): A condition characterized by an uncomfortable feeling, such as an urge to move, that is usually in the legs, gets worse when resting, gets worse later in the day, and gets better when you're up and moving that isn't better explained by any other disease or condition.

Ropinirole: A medication in the dopamine agonist class, frequently used to treat RLS and Parkinson's disease.

Schedules: The organization system used by the Drug Enforcement Agency to stratify the risk of medications to be abused or diverted.

Sclerotherapy: A treatment for varicose veins that involves injecting a chemical into the veins to make them shrink.

Seizures: Uncontrolled electrical activity in the brain leading to abnormal behaviors or sensations.

Selective serotonin reuptake inhibitors (SSRIs): A class of medications frequently used to treat depression or anxiety.

Sensorimotor disorder: A condition in which uncomfortable sensations lead to movements; the sensations are the primary disorder rather than the movements, but both unpleasant sensations and excessive movement are often present together.

Sequential compression device: A machine that squeezes the legs.

Serotonin: A chemical messenger in the brain with a variety of functions including mood regulation.

Serotonin and norepinephrine reuptake inhibitors (SNRIs): A class of medications frequently used to treat depression or pain.

Shingles: A painful skin condition caused by the herpes zoster virus.

Sickle cell disease: A group of genetic diseases that affect the body's ability to make healthy red blood cells.

Sleep study: The informal term for polysomnography.

Sleep-onset myoclonus: Also known as sleep-onset myoclonus, these are sudden, brief jerking movements that occur just prior to falling asleep.

Small-fiber nerves: Specialized nerves that are responsible for transmitting signals from the body to the brain regarding pain and temperature sensation and controlling the automatic functions of the body, such as digestion, heart rate, and sweating.

Small-fiber neuropathy: Damaged or disordered small-fiber nerves.

Small intestinal bacterial overgrowth (SIBO): A condition characterized by excessive small intestinal bacteria thought to cause diarrhea or poor absorption of nutrients.

Sodium channel blocker: A class of medications frequently used to reduce seizures.

Spinal tap: Also known as a lumbar puncture, a spinal tap is a medical procedure performed by inserting a needle into the low back to remove the fluid that surrounds the brain and spinal cord.

Stevens-Johnson syndrome: A severe reaction to a medication that consists of painful, raw, blistering, and peeling skin.

Stroke: Permanent damage done to the brain due to either a loss of blood flow or bleeding into the brain.

Suggested immobilization test (SIT): A test for RLS that requires participants to sit still for 60 minutes and report the severity of their symptoms during the course of the test.

Syndrome: A group of symptoms that occur together.

Tactile: Related to the sense of touch.

Telehealth: Interactions between providers and patients that take place using telecommunications; can be voice only or voice and video.

Test dose: A small dose of a medicine used to assess for any allergic reactions prior to administration of the full dose.

Testosterone: The primary hormone responsible for generating male sexual characteristics.

Tetracyclic: A class of medications frequently used to treat depression.

Tetrahydrocannabinol (THC): The primary psychoactive chemical in cannabis.

Third trimester: The portion of pregnancy that begins at week 28 and ends at childbirth.

Thyroid hormone: A hormone made in the thyroid gland that contributes to the regulation of chemical reactions in the body known as metabolism.

Tolerance: Deriving less benefit from the same dose of a medication or substance.

Tonic motor activation (TOMAC) system: A device that uses electrical stimulation of the nerves in the legs to treat RLS.

Toxicity: Harmful consequences from excessively high blood levels of a medication or substance.

Transcutaneous electrical nerve stimulation (TENS) unit: A device that uses electrical stimulation to cause muscle contractions.

Transferrin: A protein that binds to and transports iron in the blood.

Transferrin saturation: The percentage of transferrin in the blood that is attached to iron. This is calculated by taking the amount of iron in the blood and dividing by the amount of transferrin. Lower values indicate potential deficiency.

Ultrasound: A medical procedure that uses sound waves to create images of the body.

Unconscious: The absence of intentional thought.

Varicose veins: Large, twisted veins that are typically visible just under the skin.

Vascular resistance: The degree of constriction in the arteries that controls blood pressure.

Vascular surgery: A field of medicine devoted to the treatment of diseases of arteries, veins, and lymphatic vessels.

Veins: Tubes for moving blood toward the heart.

Vitamin D: A compound synthesized in the skin when exposed to sunlight and used by the body in numerous chemical reactions, also sold as a dietary supplement.

Vitamin D deficiency: Inadequate levels of vitamin D in the blood.

Vulnerable: A term for people who are at greater risk of developing a disease or obtaining inadequate health care.

Willis-Ekbom disease: Another name for RLS. Sir Thomas Willis described RLS in 1672. Karl-Axel Ekbom brought the condition to modern consciousness in 1945.

RESOURCES AND FURTHER READING

Government

Substance Abuse and Mental Health Services (SAMHSA)
Call 1-800-662-HELP (4357) for 24/7 confidential information for substance use and mental health concerns or visit FindTreatment.gov.
Suicide and Crisis Lifeline: Call 988
Opioid Risk Tool: https://nida.nih.gov/sites/default/files/opioidrisktool.pdf
Sample opioid pain agreement: https://www.fda.gov/files/drugs/publis hed/Opioid-Patient-Prescriber-Agreement-(PPA).pdf

Foundations and Societies

The Restless Legs Syndrome Foundation is a great source of up-to-date, trustworthy medical information for patients and loved ones. They sponsor research and advocacy events. They publish a quarterly magazine called *NightWalkers* to provide ongoing updates to its members. Membership costs are low and allow access to additional information. Visit www.rls.org.

The Restless Legs Syndrome Foundation also releases information for health care providers that some patients might be interested in reviewing, including "The Management of Restless Legs Syndrome: An Updated Algorithm" by Dr. Michael Silber and colleagues published in July 2021. This article can be accessed using common search engines.

The American Academy of Sleep Medicine (AASM) sponsors www.sle epeducation.org, a website that provides information about many sleep disorders, including RLS.

The International Restless Legs Society Study Group (IRLSSG) uses a rating scale to determine the severity of RLS, particularly for use during research on RLS. This scale can be found here: https://biolincc.nhlbi.nih.gov/media/studies/masm/IRLS.pdf?link_time=2019-07-07_21:09:19.282153.

Mental Health America offers a free screening test for depression here: https://screening.mhanational.org/screening-tools/depression/.

Health Care Provider–Sponsored Patient Information

For information about prescription drugs and supplements, Mayo Clinic offers a helpful website: https://www.mayoclinic.org/drugs-supplements/. You can review your medications and possible side effects here.

Dr. Andy Berkowksi of ReLACS Health operates a telemedicine-based direct specialty care sleep medicine practice with special expertise in RLS management. His blog provides insight into topics about RLS that are often overlooked elsewhere. It can be found on his website: www.relacshealth.com.

Dr. Chris Winter does a terrific podcast on everything related to sleep. It's called Sleep Unplugged, and I highly recommend following it. Episode 13 is about RLS, and it's well worth the 39 minutes to listen to it.

If reading this book wasn't enough and you want to hear me talk to my colleagues about RLS, you can watch a video of a lecture I gave to the Duke Department of Neurology on February 1, 2023, here: https://www.youtube.com/watch?v=jYvc5_SrbBE (starts at 14:30). The talk is titled "Breaking the Addiction: Moving Beyond Dopamine Agonists for the Treatment of Restless Legs Syndrome."

ABOUT *BRAIN & LIFE* AND THE AMERICAN ACADEMY OF NEUROLOGY

Brain & Life˙ is the only magazine and website focused on the intersection of brain health and neurologic disease. A print subscription to *Brain & Life* (six issues a year) is available for free to anyone residing in the United States. Visit BrainandLife.org to subscribe or read stories on brain science, brain health and wellness, and living well with neurologic disorders.

Brain & Life is an official publication of the American Academy of Neurology (AAN). Founded in 1948, the AAN represents more than 36,000 members who are neurologists and neuroscience professionals and is dedicated to promoting the highest-quality patient-centered neurologic care. A neurologist is a doctor with specialized training in diagnosing, treating, and managing disorders of the brain and nervous system such as Alzheimer's disease, stroke, migraine, multiple sclerosis, concussion, Parkinson's disease, and epilepsy. For more information about the American Academy of Neurology, visit AAN.com.

INDEX

For the benefit of digital users, indexed terms that span two pages (e.g., 52–53) may, on occasion, appear on only one of those pages

Figures and tables are indicated by *f* and *t* following the page number.

AAN (American Academy of Neurology), 237
AASM (American Academy of Sleep Medicine), 128–29, 235
abuse, 211, 108
access to care, 184
accommodations, 198
acetaminophen, 118
  definition of, 211
  premedication for iron therapy, 64
acupuncture, 211, 81
acute inflammation, 211, 203
addiction (dependence), 108
  definition of, 215, 192
  monitoring for, 192
adenosine, 211, 32, 33, 203, 208
ADHD (attention deficit hyperactivity disorder), 50, 164–65
adrenal gland, 211
advocacy, 194

Aggrenox (dipyridamole with aspirin), 138
agonists, 211
air hunger, 211
akathisia, 11–12
  definition of, 211
  drug-induced, 11–12, 12*t*
alcohol, 26
allergies, 167–68
alpha-2-delta ligands. *See* gabapentinoids
alpha-2-delta receptors, 211, 101
alprazolam, 49
  dosing, 129*t*
  duration of action, 129–30, 130*t*
amantadine, 145
American Academy of Neurology (AAN), 237
American Academy of Sleep Medicine (AASM), 128–29, 235
amitriptyline, 25*t*, 46

amphetamines, 165
antianxiety medications, 25*t*
antidepressants
    for anxiety, 49–50
    definition of, 212
    for depression, 46–48, 144, 208
    that exacerbate RLS, 25*t*, 26
antihistamines
    for akathisia, 12
    definition of, 212
    in hospitalized patients, 156
    premedication for iron
        therapy, 64
    that do not worsen RLS, 167–68
    that exacerbate RLS, 25*t*, 26,
        149, 156
anti-itching medications, 25*t*
anti–motion sickness
    medications, 25*t*
antinausea medications
    definition of, 212
    in hospitalized patients, 156
    that exacerbate RLS, 24, 25*t*, 156
antipsychotics
    definition of, 212
    that exacerbate RLS, 24, 25*t*
antiseizure drugs, 139–44
antiviral medications, 145
anxiety, 48–50
    definition of, 212
    generalized anxiety
        disorder, 217, 49
arteries, 212
asterixis, 212, 105
attention deficit hyperactivity
    disorder (ADHD),
        50, 164–65
    definition of, 212
    vignette, 165

augmentation
    definition of, 212
    with dopamine agonists, 93–
        94, 150–51
    vignettes, 191–92
autoimmune diseases, 212, 18
autonomic functions, 212

benzodiazepines (benzos), 127–34
    for anxiety, 49
    complications, 131–33,
        158–59
    definition of, 212
    discontinuation, 133–34
    dosing, 129–31, 129*t*
    duration of action, 130*t*
    history, 127–29
    in hospitalized patients, 156–57
    overdose, 132–33
    prescribing, 129–31
    side effects, 131, 159
    vignette, 130–31, 133
    while breastfeeding, 153–54
    withdrawal, 133–34
    withdrawal symptoms, 132
benzodiazepine use disorder,
        212, 134
bias, 183, 184
biopsy, 213, 9
bisexual or transgender
        patients, 183
black box warnings, 213, 64–65
blood-brain barrier, 213, 19–
        20, 21*f*
blood pressure
    high, 41–42
    low, 95
    nocturnal dip, 40–41
blood vessels, 213

brain
changes that lead to RLS, 33, 34*f*
fundamentals of structure and function of, 30–33
brain iron deficiency, 213, 17, 55
Brain & Life Books series, ix–x
Brain & Life magazine, 237
breastfeeding, 153–54
bromocriptine, 213, 87
buprenorphine
dosing and prescribing, 115*t*, 116, 118
duration of action, 117*t*
in hospitalized patients, 157–58
monitoring, 191
potency, 116–17
side effects, 120
buprenorphine/naloxone (Suboxone), 32–33, 118
bupropion, 26, 46–47, 136*t*, 144

caffeine, 26
cannabidiol (CBD), 213, 78
cannabis (marijuana), 213, 78
carbamazepine, 136*t*, 139–41, 145
carbidopa, 87
carbidopa/levodopa (Sinemet), 213, 86*t*, 87
carbohydrates, 75
cardiovascular disease, 38, 39–40, 42
cardiovascular drugs, 137–39
caregivers
information for, 187–99
vignettes, 187–88, 190–91
causes of RLS, 29–35
changes in the brain, 33, 34*f*
identifying, 188–89
unanswered questions, 201–5

CBD (cannabidiol), 213, 78
CBT-I (cognitive-behavioral therapy for insomnia), 214, 162
central sleep apnea, 213, 122–23
chelated iron, 213, 58
chemical sensitivity, 168
chlorpheniramine, 25*t*
chlorpromazine, 12*t*, 25*t*
chronic inflammation, 213, 202–3
chronic opioid therapy
common rules for, 114
See also opioids
circadian disorders, 213, 204
circadian rhythms, 213, 204
citalopram, 12*t*, 25*t*, 46
classical conditioning, 213, 162
clinical diagnosis, 214
clinical trials, 214
clonazepam, 128–29
dosing and prescribing, 129*t*, 131
duration of action, 130*t*
vignettes, 130–31, 133, 159
clonidine, 136*t*, 137–38
for ADHD, 165
doses, 137
low-dose, 137
in pregnancy, 151
side effects, 137
vignette, 145
codeine
dosing and prescribing, 115*t*, 118
duration of action, 117*t*
monitoring, 191
potency, 116–17
cognitive-behavioral therapy for insomnia (CBT-I), 214, 162

cognitive disabilities, patients with, 183–84
colonoscopy, 214, 68–69
coma, 214, 132–33
combination pills, 118
compression, 73
compression devices, sequential (pneumatic), 73–74
compression stockings, 214, 74
compulsive behaviors
   drug-induced, 53
   monitoring for, 190–91
   vignette, 190–91
compulsive gambling, 92, 97
computed tomography (CT) scan, 215
conditioning, classical, 213, 162
conditions that mimic RLS, 7–12
confidentiality, 193
consequences of RLS, 37–54
constipation, 119
continuous positive airway pressure (CPAP) machine, 214, 122, 162–63
controlled substances, 214, 108–9, 179
copays, 214, 180–81
coronary artery disease, 214
correlation without causation, 214, 38
corticosteroids
   definition of, 214
   premedication for iron therapy, 64
cortisol, 214, 41
costs, 180–81
counterstimulation, 215, 72–74
COVID-19, 215, 168–69
COVID-associated RLS, 168–69

CPAP (continuous positive airway pressure) machine, 214, 122, 162–63
cramps, nighttime, 11
Crohn's disease, 215, 202–3
CT (computed tomography) scan, 215
cystic fibrosis, 215, 181–82

DaT (dopamine transporter) scans, 216, 205
DAWS (dopamine agonist withdrawal syndrome), 215, 95–96
daytime sleepiness, 51–52
DEA (Drug Enforcement Agency), 108
delirium, 132
dementia, 50
   definition of, 215
   special considerations for people with, 158–60
   vignette, 159
demographics, 16–17
dependence (addiction), 108
   definition of, 215, 192
   monitoring for, 192
depression, 42–49
   definition of, 215
   monitoring for, 191
   screening test for, 236
   vignettes, 43, 45
devices, 78–81
diabetes, 215
diagnosis, 3–5, 174–75
   clinical, 214
   confirming, 13
   in dementia patients, 160
   unanswered questions, 205–7

diagnostic criteria, 3–4
dialysis, 215, 21–22
diaphragm, 215
diazepam
  for anxiety, 49
  dosing, 129t
  duration of action, 129–30, 130t
dietary interventions, 75–76, 209
  vignette, 75
dietary iron, 56, 57t
dietary supplements, 75–78
dimenhydrinate, 25t
diphenhydramine
  for akathisia, 12
  side effects, 25t, 26, 156
  vignettes, 147, 149
dipyridamole, 136t, 138–39
  doses, 138
  future directions, 208
  in pregnancy, 151
  vignette, 139, 145
dipyridamole with aspirin
  (Aggrenox), 138
disabilities, people with, 183–84
distraction, 74–75, 189
diuretics, 215, 106
diversion, 215
dopamine, 215, 24, 30–31, 33, 165
dopamine agonists, 31, 85–97, 86t,
  150–51, 193
  augmentation from, 208–9
  complications, 91–94, 210
  for dementia patients, 159
  discontinuation, 95–97
  dosage, 88–89, 89t, 93–94
  future directions, 208–9
  history of, 86–88
  for hospitalized
    patients, 157–58

monitoring, 190
in pregnancy, 150–51
side effects, 90–91, 167,
  190, 197
vignette, 88, 89, 91, 92, 94, 97
while breastfeeding, 153
withdrawal, 95–97
dopamine agonist withdrawal
  syndrome (DAWS),
  215, 95–96
dopamine antagonists, 25t
dopamine receptors, 31
dopamine therapy. See dopamine
  agonists
dopamine transporter (DaT)
  scans, 216, 205
doxylamine, 25t
Drug Enforcement Agency
  (DEA), 224, 108
drug testing, 114–15
Duke Department of
  Neurology, 236
duloxetine, 25t, 46
dysesthesia, 216, 2

ECG or EKG (electrocardiogram),
  216, 121
edema, peripheral, 222, 106
electrocardiogram (ECG or EKG),
  216, 121
electromyogram (EMG), 9, 182
elemental iron, 216, 60–61
EMG (electromyogram), 9, 182
epilepsy, 216
escitalopram, 25t, 46
estrogen, 216, 149
ethnic minority
  populations, 181–83
excitatory neurotransmitters, 30

exercise, 82–83, 189, 209
  vignettes, 113
experimental therapies, 209

fatigue, 216, 95
ferric carboxymaltose
  definition of, 216
  dosing and recommendations
    for use, 63t
  intravenous (IV)
    infusions, 62–63
ferric citrate
  definition of, 216
  oral supplements, 57–58
ferric sulfate
  definition of, 216
  oral supplements, 57–58
ferritin
  choosing between oral and IV
    iron 67
  definition of, 216
  lab tests, 18–19, 20f, 55–56
  unanswered questions, 206–7
  vignettes, 68, 182
ferrous fumarate
  definition of, 216
  oral supplements, 57–58
ferrous gluconate
  definition of, 216
  oral supplements, 57–58, 60–61
ferrous sulfate
  definition of, 217
  oral supplements, 57–58, 60–61
  vignette, 175
ferumoxytol
  black box warning, 64–65
  definition of, 217
  dosing and recommendations
    for use, 63t

intravenous (IV)
  infusions, 62–63
fexofenadine, 26, 156, 167–68
fibromyalgia, 217
FindTreatment.gov, 235
flumazenil, 133
fluoxetine, 12t, 25t, 46
fluphenazine, 25t
fMRI (functional MRI),
  217, 205–6
folate (vitamin B9), 217, 148–49
folic acid, 148–49
food(s)
  food triggers, 75
  recommended foods to eat
    and to avoid when taking
    nonheme iron supplements,
    59, 59t
  that reduce inflammation, 76
functional MRI (fMRI),
  217, 205–6
future directions, 207–9

GABA (gamma-aminobutyric
    acid), 217, 101, 127–28
gabapentin, extended-release
  (Gralise), 100
gabapentin (Neurontin), 99–
  100, 100t
  complications, 107
  definition of, 217
  discontinuation and
    withdrawal, 109–10
  dosing, 102–3, 104t
  in hospitalized patients, 156–57
  in pregnancy, 150
  side effects, 107
  vignettes, 101, 104, 113,
    152, 154

gabapentin enacarbil (Horizant),
    100, 100*t*
  copays, 180–81
  definition of, 217
  dosing, 103, 104*t*
  side effects, 107
  vignette, 106
gabapentinoids, 99–110, 100*t*, 193
  complications, 107–9, 158–
    59, 168
  definition of, 217
  for dementia patients, 159
  discontinuation and
    withdrawal, 109–10
  dosing, 102–5, 104*t*
  future directions, 207
  history, 99–102
  for hospitalized
    patients, 157–58
  monitoring, 191
  in pregnancy, 150, 151
  side effects, 105–7, 167, 191
  vignette, 101, 104, 106, 109
  while breastfeeding, 153
gambling, compulsive, 92, 97
gamma-aminobutyric acid
    (GABA), 217, 101, 127–28
gastroparesis, 217, 24–26
gay, lesbian, bisexual, or
    transgender patients, 183
gender minorities, 183
generalized anxiety disorder,
    217, 49
generic medications, 217
genes, 217
genetics
  definition of, 218
  predisposition for RLS, 27
  unanswered questions, 201–2

gestational RLS, 148
glia, 218, 30
glutamate, 32, 33, 203
Gralise (gabapentin, extended-
    release), 100
gynecologists, 218, 194

half-life, 218, 117–18
hallucinations, 218, 90
haloperidol, 12*t*, 25*t*
health care costs, 180–81
health conditions that contribute
    to RLS, 21–24
health insurance, 180–81, 185
heart attack risk, 39–40
heart disease, 22–23, 38–42
heart failure, 218, 16–17, 23
heat therapy, 72–73
hematologists, 218, 63
heme iron, 218, 56
heme iron supplements, 58
hemochromatosis, 218, 65–66
herbal supplements, 77–78
heroin, 32–33
high blood pressure, 41–42
high-molecular-weight (HMW)
    iron dextran, 218, 62
Horizant. *See* gabapentin
    enacarbil
hormones, 218
hospitalized patients, 156–58
  vignette, 157
hot water therapy, 72
hydrocodone
  dosing and prescribing, 115*t*, 118
  duration of action, 117*t*
  monitoring, 191
  potency, 116–17
hydrocodone/acetaminophen, 118

hydromorphone, 157
hydroxyzine, 25*t*
hypertension, 41–42
hypnic jerks, 218, 10
hypotension, 95

ICDs. *See* impulse control disorders
ice baths, 72–73
immune system disorders, 167–68
impulse control disorders (ICDs)
    definition of, 218
    drug-induced, 92–93, 96
    eating-related, 167
    monitoring for, 190–91
inattention, 219, 164
inflammation
    acute, 211, 203
    chronic, 213, 202–3
    unanswered questions, 202–3
infrared light therapy, 209
inhibitory neurotransmitters, 30
insomnia, 44, 160
    cognitive-behavioral therapy
        for insomnia (CBT-I), 162
    definition of, 219
    with RLS, 161–62, 163*f*
    sleep disorders, 160–64
    treatment of, 46, 162, 163*f*
    vignette, 160–61
International Restless Legs Society
    Study Group (IRLSSG) rating
    scale, 236
intravenous (IV) iron infusions,
    62–66, 69
    choosing between oral iron
        and, 66–68
    dosing and recommendations
        for use, 62–63, 63*t*
    vignettes, 175, 182

IRLSSG (International Restless
    Legs Society Study Group)
    rating scale, 236
iron
    chelated, 213, 58
    definition of, 213
    dietary, 56, 57*t*
    elemental, 216, 60–61
    heme, 218, 56
    nonheme, 221, 56, 58–59
iron deficiency, 16–20, 33, 55, 210
    brain, 213
    definition of, 219
    diagnosis of, 206–7
iron dextran
    high-molecular-weight
        (HMW), 218, 62–63
    low-molecular-weight (LMW),
        220, 62–65, 63*t*, 66, 68
iron gluconate
    dosing and recommendations
        for use, 63*t*
    intravenous (IV)
        infusions, 62–63
iron infusion reaction, 219, 65
iron infusions. *See* intravenous
    (IV) iron infusions
iron isomaltoside
    definition of, 219
    dosing and recommendations
        for use, 63*t*
    intravenous (IV) infusions,
        62–63, 66
iron sucrose
    definition of, 219
    dosing and recommendations
        for use, 63*t*
    intravenous (IV)
        infusions, 62–63

iron supplements, 57–62, 69
    doses, 60–61
    recommended foods to eat and
        to avoid when taking, 59, 59t
    vignettes, 59–60, 149, 166
iron tests
    algorithm for understanding
        results, 19, 20f
    interpreting, 15, 55–56, 206–7
iron therapy, 55–69
    additional, 68–69
    for dementia patients, 159, 160
    follow-up testing, 68–69
    intravenous (IV) infusions, 62–
        68, 63t, 69
    oral, 57–62, 66–68
    premedication, 64
    vignettes, 20, 59–60, 61, 68,
        175, 182

jerks, hypnic, 218, 10

kidney disease, 219, 16–17,
    21–22, 44
kidney failure, 22

labeling, 174–75
lamotrigine, 136t, 143–44, 151
large-fiber nerves, 219
large-fiber neuropathy, 219, 9
lasers, 209
leg cramps, nighttime, 11
lesbian, bisexual, or transgender
    patients, 183
levetiracetam, 136t, 143
levodopa, 87
limb movement arousal, 219, 173–74
LMW iron dextran. See low-
    molecular-weight iron dextran

long COVID-19, 219, 168–69
long QT syndrome, 219, 121
loratadine, 156, 167–68
lorazepam, 49
    dosing, 129t
    duration of action, 130t
loved ones
    how RLS affects, 194–98
    information for, 187–99
    vignettes, 187–88, 190–91, 195, 197
low blood pressure, 220, 95
low-income populations, 184
    urban, 180–81
    vignette, 180
low-molecular-weight (LMW)
        iron dextran
    definition of, 220
    dosing and recommendations
        for use, 63t
    intravenous (IV) infusions,
        62–65, 66
    vignettes, 68
Lyrica. See pregabalin

magnesium, 220, 76
magnetic resonance imaging
        (MRI), 66
    definition of, 220
    functional (fMRI), 217, 205–6
marijuana (cannabis), 213, 78
massage, 73, 189
mast cell activation syndrome
        (MCAS), 220, 168
Mayo Clinic resources, 236
MCAS (mast cell activation
        syndrome), 220, 168
meclizine, 25t
medical conditions that mimic
    RLS, 7–12

medications
  additional, 135–46
  benzodiazepines (benzos), 212,
    127–34, 129*t*, 130*t*, 153–54
  booster doses, 197
  cardiovascular drugs, 137–39
  combination pills, 118
  costs, 180–81
  dopamine agonists, 31, 85–97,
    86*t*, 153
  future directions, 207–
    8, 209–10
  gabapentinoids, 217, 99–110,
    100*t*, 150, 151, 153
  in hospitalized patients, 156
  iron therapy, 55–69
  monitoring, 189–93
  off-label, 221, 135–36
  opioids, 111–25, 115*t*,
    117*t*, 153–54
  for PLMD, 175–76
  in pregnancy, 150–52
  premedication, 223
  prescription drug
    resources, 236
  side effects, 15, 53
  test doses, 226, 63–64
  that cause akathisia, 11–12,
    12*t*
  that cause RLS, 24–27, 25*t*
  uncommonly used prescription
    drugs, 135–36, 136*t*
  vignettes, 145, 154
  See also specific medications
melatonin, 220, 204
Mental Health America screening
  test for depression, 236
methadone
  complications, 123

dosing and prescribing, 115*t*, 116
  duration of action, 117*t*
  in hospitalized patients, 157
  monitoring, 191
  potency, 116–17
  side effects, 120
  vignettes, 123, 139, 145,
    157, 191–92
methylphenidate, 165
metoclopramide, 24–26, 25*t*
migraine, 220
MiraLAX (polyethylene glycol), 119
Mirapex. *See* pramipexole
mirtazapine, 25*t*, 46
morning symptoms, 92, 93
morphine
  complications, 168
  dosing, 115*t*
  duration of action, 117*t*
  monitoring, 191
  potency, 116–17
MRI. *See* magnetic resonance
  imaging
MR spectroscopy, 220, 205–6
MS. *See* multiple sclerosis
multiple chemical sensitivity,
  220, 168
multiple sclerosis (MS), 220, 16–
  17, 23
mu-opioid receptor, 112
myoclonus, 10–11
  definition of, 220
  drug-induced, 119–20
  sleep-onset, 225, 10
  vignette, 10

naloxone (Narcan), 121–22
narcolepsy, 220, 160
narcotics, 220, 112

near-infrared light therapy, 78–79
definition of, 220
vignette, 79
nerve conduction studies, 221, 9
nerves, 220
Neupro. *See* rotigotine
neurologists, 221, 17
neurons, 221, 30
Neurontin. *See* gabapentin
neuropathy, 7–9
brief overview, 9
large-fiber, 219, 9
peripheral, 223, 7–8, 21,
33–34
small-fiber, 225, 9
vignette, 8
neurotransmitters, 24
definition of, 221
excitatory, 30
inhibitory, 30
unanswered questions, 203–4
nighttime leg cramps, 11
NightWalkers, 235
nocturnal dip, 221, 40–41
nonheme iron, 221, 56, 58–59
nonheme iron supplements
foods that are recommended
to eat and to avoid when
taking, 59*t*
oral supplements, 59
nonpharmacological options, 209
norepinephrine, 221, 137
nortriptyline, 25*t*
numbness, 8–9

obesity, 166–67
definition of, 221
vignettes, 166
obstetricians, 221

obstructive sleep apnea (OSA),
160, 162–64
definition of, 221
vignette, 5
off-label medications, 221, 135–36
older adults, 159–60
ondansetron, 156
opiates, 221, 111–12
opioid contracts, 114, 235
vignette, 123
opioid reversal agents, 121–22
Opioid Risk Tool, 221, 113–
14, 235
opioids, 111–25, 117*t*, 191–92, 193
bias and stigma to, 183, 184–85
common rules for chronic
opioid therapy, 114
complications, 120–23, 168
for dementia patients, 159
discontinuation and
withdrawal, 124–25
dosing, 115–19, 115*t*, 122
endogenous, 32–33
history, 111–15
for hospitalized patients, 156–
57, 158
monitoring, 192–93
in pregnancy, 150, 151
prescribing, 115–19
side effects, 119–20
unanswered questions, 203–4
vignettes, 118–19, 139, 157
while breastfeeding, 153–54
withdrawal, 124–25
withdrawal symptoms, 121
opioid use disorder (OUD),
113, 121
definition of, 221
vignette, 32–33

opium, 222, 111–12
oral iron supplements, 57–62
  choosing between IV iron
    and, 66–68
  vignette, 59–60, 61
OSA. *See* obstructive sleep
  apnea
other sleep disorders, 160–64
OUD. *See* opioid use disorder
oxcarbazepine, 136*t*, 141
oxycodone, 32
  complications, 123, 168
  definition of, 222
  dosing, 115*t*
  duration of action, 117*t*
  monitoring, 191
  potency, 116–17
oxygen levels, 34

pain, 2–3, 8
painful legs moving toes
  syndrome, 222, 12
pain medications that exacerbate
  RLS, 25*t*
pandemics, 222
panic attacks, 222, 127–28
panic disorder, 222, 49
Parkinson's disease, 30–31
  definition of, 222
  vignette, 30–31
paroxetine, 12*t*, 25*t*, 46
pergolide, 222, 87
periodic limb movement disorder
  (PLMD), 6
  definition of, 222
  diagnosis of, 173–74
  labeling, 174–75
  vs PLMS, 173–74
  treatment of, 175–76

periodic limb movement (PLM)
  index, 222, 5–6
periodic limb movements, 171–76
periodic limb movements of
  sleep (PLMS), 5–7, 40, 171–
    73, 196–97
  definition of, 222, 174
  labeling, 174–75
  vs PLMD, 173–74
  vignettes, 172, 173
periodic limb movements of wake
  (PLMW), 222, 5–6
peripheral edema, 222, 106
peripheral nervous system,
  223, 33–34
peripheral neuropathy, 223, 7–
  8, 33–34
peroneal nerve, 223, 80
perphenazine, 25*t*
physical disabilities, patients
  with, 183–84
physician assistants, 223
placebos, 223, 78–79
PLMD. *See* periodic limb
  movement disorder
PLM (periodic limb movement)
  index, 222, 5–6
PLMS. *See* periodic limb
  movements of sleep
PLMW (periodic limb movements
  of wake), 222, 5–6
PM medications, 26
pneumatic compression devices,
  223, 73–74
polyethylene glycol
  (MiraLAX), 119
polysomnography (PSG), 223, 4–5
potency, 223, 116–17
pramipexole (Mirapex), 86*t*, 87

common doses, 89*t*
complications, 92–94
definition of, 223
in hospitalized patients, 156–57
side effects, 90
vignettes, 88, 89, 91, 92, 94, 97,
    113, 118–19, 123, 139, 178–
    79, 190–92
precision medicine, 208
pregabalin (Lyrica), 100, 100*t*
complications, 107, 108–9
definition of, 223
dosing, 103–5, 104*t*
in hospitalized patients, 156–57
in pregnancy, 150
side effects, 107, 167
vignettes, 106, 109, 113
pregnancy, 147–54
medications during, 150–
    52, 154
RLS after, 152–53, 194
RLS during, 148–49
third trimester, 226, 148, 149
vignettes, 149, 152, 154, 194
premedication, 223
prenatal vitamins, 223, 148–49
prescription drugs
combination pills, 118
controlled substances, 179
half-life, 117–18
resources, 236
uncommonly used, 135–
    36, 136*t*
See also medications; *specific
    medications*
prior authorization, 223, 180–81
prochlorperazine, 12*t*
progesterone, 224, 149
prolactin, 224, 149

promethazine, 12*t*, 25*t*, 156
proprietary blends, 224
proprietary supplements, 77–78
PSG (polysomnography), 223, 4–5

QT interval
definition of, 224
long QT syndrome, 219, 121

racial and ethnic minority
    populations, 181–83
rating scale (IRLSSG), 236
rebound RLS, 224, 117
receptors, 224
refractory RLS, 113
definition of, 224
vignette, 113
ReLACS Health resources, 236
relapses, 224, 134
relationship discord, 52–53
vignette, 52–53
relearning to sleep, 162, 163*f*
repetitive transcranial magnetic
    stimulation (rTMS),
    224, 80–81
Requip. *See* ropinirole
research
clinical trials, 214
future directions, 209–10
resources
foundations and
    societies, 235–36
government, 235
health care provider–sponsored
    patient information, 236
information for loved ones and
    caregivers, 187–99
respiratory depression, 224, 121
Restiffic, 224, 74

restless legs syndrome (RLS), xi
  alternative theories of, 33–35
  overview, 1–13
  causes of, 29–35, 188–89, 201–5
  conditions that mimic, 7–12
  confirming your diagnosis, 13
  consequences of, 37–54
  contributing health
    conditions, 21–24
  COVID-associated, 168–69
  definition of, 224
  diagnosis, 3–5, 174–75, 205–7
  vs drug-induced
    akathisia, 11–12
  gestational, 148
  identifying causes of, 188–89
  labeling, 174–75
  medication triggers, 24–27, 25t
  vs neuropathy, 7–9
  vs nighttime leg cramps, 11
  with other illnesses, 155–69
  vs painful legs moving toes
    syndrome, 12
  vs PLMS, 5–7
  prevalence of, 16, 166
  rebound, 117
  refractory, 113–14
  risk factors, 15–16
  treatment of (*see* treatment)
  typical symptoms, 1–3
  vignettes, 24–26
  in vulnerable
    populations, 177–85
Restless Legs Syndrome
  Foundation, 128–29
  Medical Advisory
    Board, 115–16
  resources, 235
risk factors, 15–16

RLS. *See* restless legs syndrome
ropinirole (Requip), 86–87, 86t
  common doses, 89t
  complications, 92–93
  definition of, 224
  in hospitalized patients, 156–57
rotigotine (Neupro), 86t, 87
  common doses, 89t
  complications, 92–93
  copays, 180–81
  in hospitalized patients, 157–58
rTMS (repetitive transcranial
    magnetic stimulation),
    224, 80–81
rural populations, 178–79, 184
  vignette, 178–79

schedules, 224
schizophrenia, 30
sclerotherapy, 224, 81–82
seizures, 225
selective serotonin reuptake
    inhibitors (SSRIs)
  for anxiety, 49–50
  definition of, 225
  that exacerbate RLS, 25t, 46
sensorimotor disorders, 225
sequential compression devices,
    225, 73–74
serotonin, 26
  definition of, 225
  unanswered questions, 203
serotonin-norepinephrine
    reuptake inhibitors (SNRIs)
  definition of, 225
  that exacerbate RLS, 25t, 46
sertraline, 25t
sexual activity, 74–75
sexual minorities, 183

shingles, 225
SIBO (small intestinal bacterial overgrowth), 225, 202–3
sickle cell disease, 225, 181–82
Sinemet. *See* carbidopa/levodopa
SIT (suggested immobilization test), 226, 4–5
sleep apnea
 central, 213, 122–23
 obstructive (OSA), 221, 5, 160, 162–64
sleep deprivation, 164, 196–97
sleepiness, daytime, 51–52
sleep medications that exacerbate RLS, 25*t*, 156
sleep-onset myoclonus, 225, 10
sleep studies, 4–5
 definition of, 225
 in dementia patients, 160
sleep testing, 4–5
Sleep Unplugged podcast, 236
sleepwalking, 51, 160
small-fiber nerves, 225
small-fiber neuropathy, 225, 9
small intestinal bacterial overgrowth (SIBO), 225, 202–3
SNRIs. *See* serotonin-norepinephrine reuptake inhibitors
sodium channel blockers, 225, 139–40
spinal tap, 226, 17
SSRIs. *See* selective serotonin reuptake inhibitors
Stevens-Johnson syndrome, 226, 140–41
stigma, 184–85
stimulants, 165

stroke, 226, 16–17, 23, 39
Suboxone. *See* buprenorphine/naloxone
Substance Abuse and Mental Health Services Administration (SAMHSA)
 FindTreatment.gov, 235
 hotline, 121, 193
 Opioid Risk Tool, 235
 resources, 235
 sample Opioid Patient Prescriber Agreement (PPA), 235
 Suicide and Crisis Lifeline, 235
suggested immobilization test (SIT), 226, 4–5
Suicide and Crisis Lifeline (SAMHSA), 235
supplements, 75–78
surgery, 23
 vascular, 227, 82
syndromes, 226

tactile counterstimulation, 73–74
teamwork, 189
telehealth, 179, 185
 definition of, 226
 vignette, 178–79
temperature counterstimulation, 72–73
TENS (transcutaneous electrical nerve stimulation), 80 227
terminology, xi, 2, 3, 101, 174–75
test doses, 226, 63–64
testosterone
 definition of, 226
 low, 122, 123
tetracyclics
 definition of, 226

that exacerbate RLS, 25*t*, 46
tetrahydrocannabinol (THC), 226, 78
thioridazine, 25*t*
third trimester, 226, 148, 149
thyroid hormone, 226, 141
TMS (transcranial magnetic stimulation), repetitive (rTMS), 224, 80–81
tobacco, 26
tolerance, 226, 91
tonic motor activation (TOMAC) system, 226, 80
topiramate, 136*t*, 142, 151
touch therapy, 73–74
toxicity, 226
Traditional Chinese Medicine, 211
tramadol
    dosing and prescribing, 115*t*, 116
    duration of action, 117*t*
    monitoring, 191
    side effects, 120
transcranial magnetic stimulation, repetitive (rTMS), 224, 80–81
transcutaneous electrical nerve stimulation (TENS), 80 227
transferrin, 227, 18–19
transferrin saturation
    choosing between oral and IV iron, 67
    definition of, 227
    lab tests, 18, 20*f*, 55–56
    unanswered questions, 206–7
    vignette, 68
transgender patients, 183
travel, 197–98
trazodone, 46

treatment
    future directions, 207–9
    iron therapy, 55–69
    for low-income urban populations, 180–81
    medications, 31, 53 (*see also* medications)
    nonpharmacological options, 209
    for racial and ethnic minority populations, 181–83
    for rural populations, 178–79
    team, 189
    vignettes, 73, 75, 88, 89, 91, 92, 94, 97, 113, 139
    without prescription drugs, 71–83
tricyclics, 25*t*

ultrasound, 227, 206
unanswered questions, 201–10
urban populations, low-income, 180–81
    vignette, 180
urine drug testing, 114–15

valproic acid, 136*t*, 142–43, 151
varicose veins, 227, 81–82
vascular resistance, 41
vascular surgery, 227, 82
venlafaxine, 25*t*, 46
vibration, 73
vignettes, 2, 5, 8, 10, 17, 20, 22, 24–26, 43, 45, 52–53, 113, 130–31, 165
vitamin B_9 (folate), 217, 148–49
vitamin C, 58–59
vitamin D, 227

vitamin D deficiency, 16–17, 23–24
    definition of, 227
    unanswered questions, 207
vitamin D supplements, 76–77
vitamins, prenatal, 223, 148–49
vulnerable populations, 227, 177–85

weighted blankets, 73
Willis-Ekbom disease (WED),
    227, xi, 3
women
    pregnant (*see* pregnancy)
    risk of heart attack, 39–40